Essential Oils to
Boost the Brain &
Heal the Body

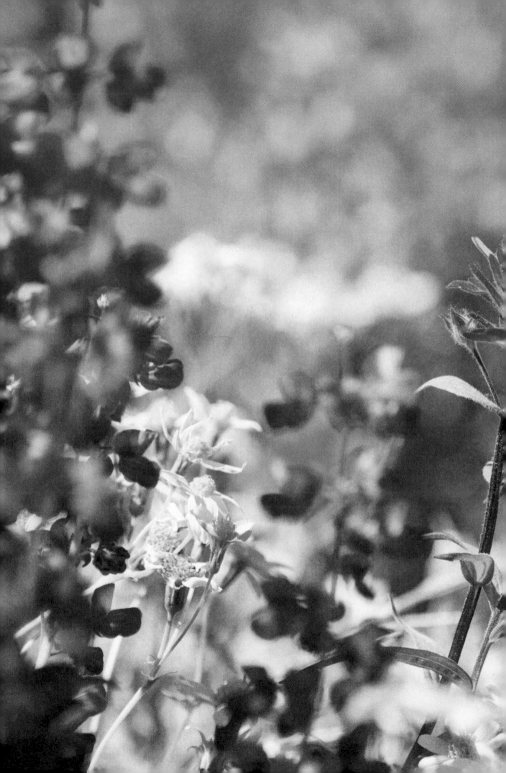

Essential Oils to Boost the Brain & Heal the Body

5 Steps to Calm Anxiety,
Sleep Better & Reduce Inflammation
to Regain Control of Your Health

Jodi Cohen

Foreword by Terry Wahls, MD

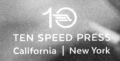

TEN SPEED PRESS
California | New York

CONTENTS

PART ONE The 5 Steps

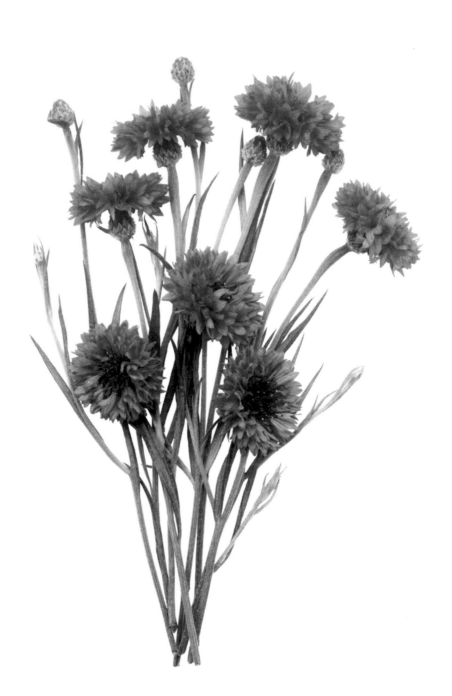

Essential oils have played a powerful role in my ability to transform lives and heal. I have been using essential oils as part of my own daily health routine since 2008. Efforts to improve my quality of sleep are what initially led me to them. I started applying chamomile and lavender before bedtime to help me relax and calm my nervous system. The oils worked so well and so immediately that I began to gradually experiment with different oils and various combinations of oils.

I recommend the use of plant-based essential oils in my best-selling book *The Wahls Protocol: A Radical Way to Treat All Chronic Autoimmune Conditions*, as I believe they contribute to the plant diversity necessary to keep you healthy. As Jodi thoroughly explains in this book, the concentrated essences of plants work on many levels, including the physical, neurological, and psychological.

Humans are meant to consume hundreds of different plant species each year, not just a handful. More diverse plant consumption adds to greater resiliency and health. As your body digests plants, thousands of metabolites (substances that are produced when the body breaks down food and chemicals) are absorbed by your gut into your bloodstream. Scientists are recognizing that these metabolites have a major impact on our risk of heart disease, autoimmune disease, mental health problems, obesity, diabetes, and even cancer. These metabolites from the digestion of a wide variety of plants contribute to how our cells do the chemistry of life. Our physiology works much better with the thousands of metabolites that come from eating a greater diversity of plants. The reality is that the food we eat is a combination of things that are incredibly good for us and a few things that are terrible for us. So, if we have variety in our diet, more diversity of foods over the week and the year, the fewer problems we will have and the more health benefits we will enjoy.

I encourage the addition of essential oils in your self-care program along with different vegetables, spices, and teas as sources of plant diversity. There are literally hundreds of essential oils and spices that you can integrate into your life to expose yourself to at least two hundred different plant species in a year.

Jodi's extensive research helps support and validate my own personal experience with essential oils, which have improved my well-being and reduced some of my subtle symptoms, like pain, headaches, constipation, and low mood. I now use cypress and frankincense most reliably, along with a blend that includes lavender, marjoram, Roman chamomile, sandalwood, vanilla, and ylang-ylang to calm my nervous system.

For self-care, my favorite ways to use essential oils are inhalation, self-massage, and in hot or ice-cold Epsom salt baths. My favorite technique involves massaging the vagus nerve and the lymphatic tissue on the sides of the neck. I start from behind my ear and massage the oils down my neck on both sides and combine that with three to five deep inhalations in each nostril before bedtime.

When I look at essential oils through a food lens, I know that essential oils are interacting positively with our biochemical pathways and nervous systems, even calming excessive inflammation. The inhalation of essential oils activates the same pathways in the brain. The topical application of essential oils on the skin ensures they are entering the bloodstream and affecting the body's pathways.

Essential Oils to Boost the Brain & Heal the Body takes these suppositions one step further, helping to explain not only how essential oils work but also the best ways to use them to combat underlying health conditions. This book is a wonderful guide for using essential oils as a powerful self-care tool to help you make steady improvements and refinements in your health.

—Terry Wahls, MD, author of *The Wahls Protocol*

Essential oils entered my life during a rock-bottom period, when no other remedies worked to calm my overwhelm, anxiety, and exhaustion. Friends gifted me a box of oils and assured me that they would help.

While I had worked with herbal remedies in my nutritional practice, my experience with essential oils was limited, as was the mental stamina required to research how and why essential oils worked. I did, however, have several years of experience as a nutritional therapist with certifications in functional neurology, yoga, and autonomic response testing that helped me understand what was happening in my own body and guide me toward the best remedy.

To be more specific, I knew that a recent prolonged stressful experience had taxed my energy reserves and tipped me into a state of intense physical and mental exhaustion, commonly referred to as adrenal fatigue. When your adrenal glands are pushed to the point of exhaustion, their ability to release the appropriate levels of the hormones necessary to fuel your energy levels is diminished. Supplements and dietary changes alone were not moving the needle, and the pharmaceutical drugs I had tried only seemed to make me feel worse.

Out of desperation, I tested the box of thirty different essential oils to determine if any of them might support my exhausted adrenal glands. I had been trained in an assessment technique known as muscle testing or asking the body questions that allow you to quickly and efficiently test many possible supplements and remedies to determine which one is best for supporting a specific physical, mental, or emotional issue. I was so depleted that I was struggling to find any remedy that tested positive.

When I used this technique to test the box of essential oils, I was both surprised and delighted when five of the oils tested well. At first, I was confused by this result, since I typically find only one or two remedies that test well. So, I pulled out the five oils—cinnamon, galbanum, manuka, rosemary, and thyme— and retested. At this point it occurred to me that I could combine them to create my own personal blend to help return my adrenal glands to balance.

At the time, I had no experience blending oils, so I just focused my intention on balancing the adrenal glands, and I muscle-tested each individual oil to determine how many drops of each to use. I combined them and then applied them directly over my adrenal glands, which are most accessible through the skin on the lower back.

Within minutes, I felt like myself for the first time in months. I had the energy to clean the house, do the laundry, go to the supermarket, and actually cook my kids' favorite meal for dinner. That night, after reading my kids to sleep, I lay awake praying for sleep myself. It then occurred to me that essential oils might offer a solution to my insomnia. I formulated another blend using the same technique of focusing on the end intention—balancing the pineal gland in the brain to release the sleep hormone melatonin and muscle-testing to find the best oils and ideal ratio—and I quickly drifted into the most restful sleep I had experienced in months.

Inspired by this early success, I began formulating additional blends to help me combat my irritability, weight gain, and fatigue. It was an intriguing experience to be both in the body of the patient and in the mind of the practitioner, where I could intellectually track how I was attempting to shift my physiology and personally experience the physical shift so immediately.

It helped me intellectually and physically understand how essential oils could be used to help shift health concerns. When my mental and physical stamina began to return, friends asked me what had helped. I began sharing my remedies with their families, friends, and clients with similar success.

With my renewed mental capacity, I began to research essential oils. I was shocked to discover that few people were using essential oil blends to support organ systems or regions of the brain. Not only that, but essential oil formulation was depicted in essential oil books and blogs to be so complicated that most people would feel unqualified to jump in.

I realized that my knowledge of physiology and my access to fellow healthcare practitioners provided immediate feedback on strategies that actually work in clinical practice. In other words, I could assess what essential oil strategies seemed to work best for most people. Across the board, when practitioners used essential oils to address the "five keys to health" that I have identified through years of trial and error, observation, and research, our clients improved.

Having personally experienced the healing power of essential oils in myself and others, I felt compelled to devote my time, energy, and passion to understanding how and why they work, a body of knowledge that I am now excited to share with you. While I would never call essential oils a miracle cure for all ailments, I do believe they can be strategically used to help your body return to balance in very specific ways that allow you to regain your health. Just as your cell phone or laptop slows down and drains the battery when too many tabs are left open, your brain fatigues when a combination of poorly functioning systems—that present as ailments—drain its energy. These stressors are additive and cumulative.

The 5 steps to healing the brain with essential oils address the five underlying energy drains that afflict most people. For some, these five strategies will return them to full health. For others, they will get them more than halfway there. But for everyone, whether healthy or health challenged, they can vastly improve their quality of life.

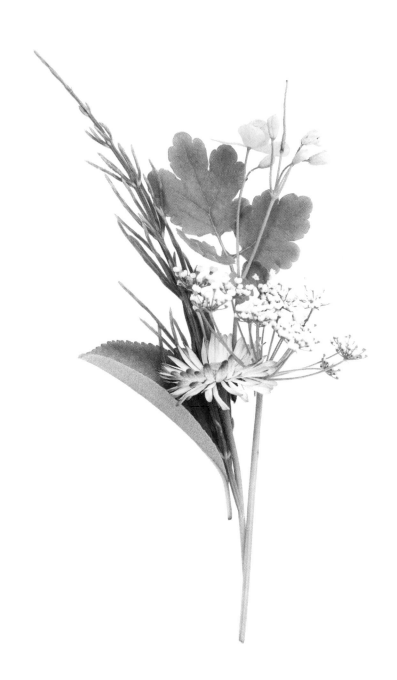

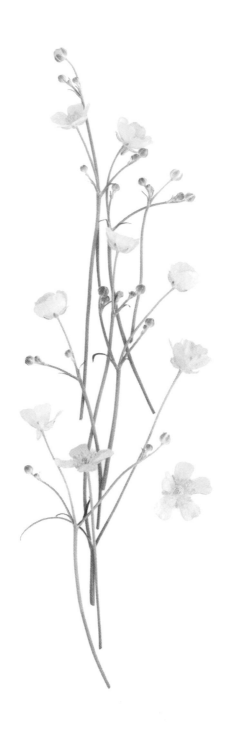

Your brain is your most important organ. It controls how you feel, how you think, how you move, and how you function. Your brain serves as the conductor—orchestrating, coordinating, and harmonizing the communication between all the systems in your body—influencing your mood, energy level, thought processes, and coordination.

Sadly, your brain might be in trouble. Dysfunction in specific parts of your brain can contribute to physical, mental, emotional, psychological, learning, or behavioral problems that present as symptoms like:

- Anxiety
- Depression
- Poor focus and concentration or difficulty learning
- Irritability
- Memory loss
- Brain fog
- Lack of motivation, drive, or passion
- Poor brain endurance (tire easily) while working, reading, or driving
- Fatigue in response to certain foods or chemicals

These symptoms impact both the elderly and the young alike, especially after any kind of head injury or concussion. What's more, these early symptoms can set in years, or even decades, before any signs of neurological disease, like Alzheimer's or Parkinson's. If you understand these early symptoms as warning signs, you can improve brain function and prevent and heal any damage.

Impacts on the Brain

Our brains are being affected by a negative synergy between many elements we consider to be commonplace:

- Poor sleep cycles
- Increased daily stress
- Rising levels of environmental toxins, including mold and heavy metals
- Blood sugar imbalances
- Chronic inflammation and immune dysregulation
- Pathogens going undetected or untreated due to misdiagnosis or ineffective treatment

All of these factors can, alone or in combination, compromise your brain's ability to process and eliminate waste products, like toxins or cellular debris. If waste is not eliminated, it can recirculate in your brain, leading to inflammation, which further compromises your protective blood-brain barrier, opening the door for more damaging material like viruses, parasites, or heavy metals to access and damage your brain. This further throws off your sleep cycles, your immune system, your hormonal balance, and your digestive function.

Here is the good news: your brain is extremely adaptable and can heal. When it comes to protecting and restoring the processes for healthy brain function, essential oils are succeeding where other remedies—and drugs—fall short.

Essential Oils Are "Essential" for Accessing the Brain

Conventional drugs have been limited in their ability to access the brain because of the blood-brain barrier, a highly selective, semi-permeable border that surrounds most of the blood vessels in the brain. These blood vessels are composed of endothelial cells wedged extremely closely together to protect the brain from potentially dangerous agents that could disturb brain function. This border prevents all but very small fat-soluble molecules from passing into the brain. The narrow space between the cells of your blood-brain barrier are known as tight junctions, which allow only those small fat-soluble molecules and some gases to pass freely through the capillary wall and into brain tissue. For this reason, it has been challenging, historically, to get the right remedy into the right region of the brain. Most conventional pharmaceuticals are neither small enough nor fat-soluble.

The molecules in essential oils are both very small and fat-soluble, allowing them to access and heal regions of the brain affected by environmental toxins and emotional and mental stress. The molecular components that make up essential oils are so small that they are known as *volatile*, meaning they easily evaporate at normal temperatures, and aromatic, meaning they circulate in the air where your nose can detect them as smell.

Why Are Essential Oils Aromatic?

The super-small size and the light weight of essential oil molecules are what make them so aromatic. They evaporate at room temperature and circulate in the air, where your nose detects them as smell. You can test this yourself: open a bottle of an oil pressed from seeds, like corn, peanut, safflower, walnut, almond, or olive, and put a few drops in a glass container. If you walk to the other side of the room, it is unlikely that you will be able to smell the seed oil. Next, repeat the experiment with an essential oil such as peppermint oil. The smell of peppermint can fill the room because the volatile molecules are airborne. It only takes one molecule of scent to communicate with the brain.

There are approximately 40 quintillion molecules in 1 drop of essential oil. (Numerically that is a 4 with 19 zeros after it: 40,000,000,000,000,000,000.) We have 100 trillion cells in our bodies, so that equates to approximately 400,000 molecules for each cell in the average human body. The vast number of molecules in 1 drop of essential oil makes them easily detected by our sense of smell.

Essential oils are also fat-soluble, which makes them especially helpful for enhancing brain function. The human brain is nearly 60 percent fat, and fat likes fat. This principle of "like attracting like" is one of the reasons that oil and water don't mix.

Fat-based bacteria, like those in your mouth, are drawn to fat-soluble remedies, like essential oils. The practice of "oil pulling"—swishing a cooking oil, like coconut oil, around in your mouth for 10 to 20 minutes—attracts the fatty membranes of bacteria to the fat in the oil like a powerful magnet. This, in effect, pulls the bacteria out of your gums into the oil, which you can then spit out. Fat-soluble essential oils are similarly drawn into your brain, where they can influence other fat-soluble hormones (sex, steroid, and thyroid hormones) to support brain health and emotional well-being.

What Are Essential Oils?

Essential oils are the natural highly concentrated essences extracted from herbs, shrubs, trees, flowers, fruits, roots, and bark in their living state. The plants from which essential oils are derived have been used for medicinal purposes throughout history. In fact, most of our modern drugs come from plants that have been modified enough to secure a patent (no natural substance can be patented). Some 50 percent of the pharmaceutical drugs produced during the last thirty years are either directly or indirectly derived from plant medicine. For example, the pain-relieving and anti-inflammatory effects of aspirin mimic the chemical compound salicin, found in white willow bark. Similarly, Valium (diazepam) is an artificial compound attempting to mimic the natural compounds found in valerian root, an herb.

Humans have long consumed plants for their healing value. Many popular healing diets consist primarily of food from organic plants and the ethically raised animals that feed on those plants. Plants, and the highly concentrated essences of plants that are distilled into essential oils, can be used to complement and support whole food healing diets and lifestyle regimens.

How Do Essential Oils Work?

Essential oils contain the key components of the plants' immune systems. They help the plants grow, thrive, evolve, and adapt to their surroundings. Oils protect plants from bacterial and viral infections, heal injuries, repel unwanted predators and other potential environmental damage, and help deliver nutrients to the cells. This makes them "essential" for a plant, since they help the plant survive. Essential oils play a similar role in the human body, perhaps due to our shared chemistry with plants. Both plants and humans are made of three primary elements—carbon, hydrogen, and oxygen—that make plants and their essential oils highly compatible with human biochemistry. Research has shown that essential oils help us fight infection (with anti-bacterial, anti-fungal, and anti-viral properties), balance hormones and emotions, and aid in regeneration.

Humans and plants both grow and thrive with a combination of sunlight, oxygen, and nutrients. Plants soak up minerals and nutrients from the soil, along with oxygen. They pass along these nutrients to us when we consume them. In *Aromatherapy for the Soul,* Valerie Ann Worwood notes, "Plants take the energy of the sun and transform it, through photosynthesis, into the food energy upon which all animals rely. Essential oils are the concentrated form of that sun energy."

The healing benefits of plants are often more accessible when the plants are immersed in water for a period of time. For example, the process of soaking and "sprouting" nuts and grains or fermenting vegetables makes the nutrients more accessible so that your body can absorb them more effectively. The same is true for the process of "steam distilling" essential oils from plants. Steam distillation exposes plants to water, heat, and pressure, making the oils contained within plant cells more accessible and therefore easier for your body to assimilate.

Essential Oils in the Brain

The blood-brain barrier is the barrier membrane between circulating blood in your body and the entrance to your brain. This membrane prevents certain damaging substances from reaching brain tissue and cerebrospinal fluid (or CSF, a clear fluid that surrounds and protects the brain), while allowing essential molecules, like oxygen and nutrients, to enter.

The blood-brain barrier is like a sieve or filter through which only molecules of a certain size or smaller can penetrate. The molecules of essential oils are so small that most of them can pass through the blood-brain barrier. Only a few substances—including gases like oxygen, carbon dioxide, alcohol, some drugs, anesthetics, and essential oils—are capable of accessing the brain in this way.

After passing through the blood-brain barrier, fat-soluble essential oil molecules easily penetrate through the cell membranes and enter brain cells, which are also composed primarily of fat. An article published in *Pharmaceuticals* called "Effect of Essential Oils on Pathogenic Bacteria," describes how essential oils easily penetrate cells and act on both the cell membrane and within the cell, "causing alterations in structure and functionality."

Your cells can't repair themselves without the proper exchange of nutrients. The ability of essential oils to increase permeability of your cell's membranes is a key reason they work to eliminate the bad bugs, like viruses and bacteria. In order to actually eliminate these pathogens, remedies need

INHALATION BYPASSES THE BLOOD-BRAIN BARRIER

Essential oils can directly access your brain through your nose.

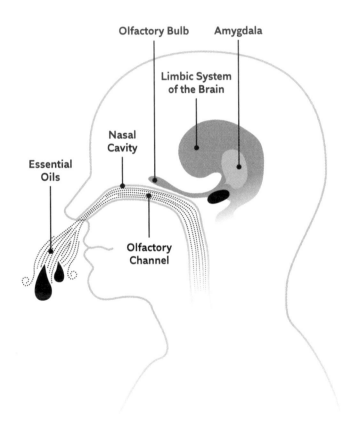

When an appropriate chemical messenger binds with cell receptors, it initiates a cascade of chemical changes inside the cells that directly impact how a person thinks, feels, and functions.

to interact with them. Certain essential oils, like those found in thyme and oregano, have been found to change the structure of the cell membrane. This, in turn, increases the permeability of the cell, allowing more nutrients in and more waste to be moved out, which accelerates healing.

In addition to increasing the permeability of cell membranes, essential oils also influence how signals are received by cell receptors that line the outside of cell membranes. These receptors receive chemical signals in the form of hormones and neurotransmitters.

Essential oils can bind to these receptor sites and activate, inhibit, or modulate the impact of other chemical messengers. For example, one of the chemical messengers that helps calm us is called GABA, which stands for gamma-aminobutyric acid. GABA is considered an inhibitory neurotransmitter because it blocks, or inhibits, certain brain signals and decreases the activity in your nervous system to help calm you down. Research has shown that a component of lavender essential oils known as linalool helps activate the calming effect of GABA.

Inhalation Bypasses Your Blood-Brain Barrier

Your sense of smell (part of your olfactory system) is the way essential oils can directly access your brain. Olfactory cells are brain cells, and the olfactory membrane in the nasal cavity is the only place in your body where the brain is directly exposed to the environment. The olfactory channel travels to the olfactory nerve, where your blood-brain barrier is the thinnest. Your blood-brain barrier is approximately eight cells in thickness across most of the brain. Around your olfactory nerve, it is only four or five cells thick. This is the reason inhalation is cited as the most efficient channel into the brain.

Once inhaled, molecules can enter the brain directly via the nasal olfactory pathway or indirectly through the circulatory system after they penetrate the lung tissue. This may help explain why anesthesia is commonly administered by inhalation.

How Your Sense of Smell Is Key to Survival

Your sense of smell is critical to survival. Smell alerts you to dangers (like predators and fire), helps track food and water, and even aids in locating certain plants for medicine. Research estimates your sense of smell to be ten thousand times more acute than your other senses.

Smell travels more quickly to the brain than your other four senses—sound, sight, taste, and touch—and has direct access to the emotional control center of the brain, known as the amygdala in your limbic system. Other senses travel to other regions of the brain first, before reaching your limbic system. This makes the sense of smell one of the most powerful avenues for targeting emotional issues such as depression or anxiety. Danger-signaling scents also keep you safe by stimulating an instinctive fear response that enables you to mobilize energy and resources quickly to survive the threat of danger.

Stop and Smell the Roses

Nobel Prize–winning researcher Linda Buck explored how different odors trigger different responses in your brain. For example, Buck found that rose essential oil can counteract your brain's fear response to predator odor. Her research found that smelling rose essential oil in the presence of predator odors (or other fear stimuli) can suppress your brain's stress responses and hormonal signals. This research gives some insight into how essential oils can influence your hormonal responses, by either suppressing or activating your brain's hormonal responses to specific odors.

The Power of Essential Oil Blends

Most research around essential oil effectiveness in balancing organ systems and regions of the brain look at combinations of certain oils (blends), not individual oils by themselves. While essential oils from individual plants are incredibly powerful, the combination of two or more oils can result in an entirely new molecular composition, where the sum is greater than the parts. This is known as a synergy between oils.

The term synergy actually means "working together in harmony." Synergy between oils is based on complex interactions among the many constituents of the individual plants from which the oils are derived, giving rise to a blend's unique characteristics and healing properties. The individual essential oils each have a multitude of compounds with beneficial, healing properties, along with weaker components that are less beneficial. Combining these individual essential oils allows one oil to balance out the weaker parts of another and even negate the possible side effects of a single oil applied on its own. For this reason, oils that might be contraindicated (not desirable) for certain conditions when used individually pose little to no threat when mixed into a blend.

Oils may work well in a blend because a compound acting alone can behave very differently in combination with other oils. For example, combining oils that are high in antimicrobial chemical components, like thymol from thyme and eugenol from clove, will create an even more effective antimicrobial remedy than just one alone.

Research by scientists on medicinal plants in *Phytotherapy Research* compared the antimicrobial activity of clove and rosemary essential oils alone and in combination and found that while "both essential oils possessed significant antimicrobial effects against all microorganisms tested [the oils in combination] indicated their additive, synergistic, or antagonistic effects against individual microorganism tests." More specifically, when the two individual oils were combined, they exerted additive antimicrobial effects against bacteria, yeast overgrowth, and mold.

Essential oil blends may also enhance the therapeutic properties of each other. For example, the anti-inflammatory effect of Roman chamomile is amplified when mixed with lavender. In addition, the anti-spasmic effects of caraway are enhanced by the anti-spasmic effects of peppermint in relieving irritable bowel syndrome (IBS) and indigestion. Blending oils creates a synergy that differs from the benefits of the individual oils, often enabling you to use less while producing better results.

This book is designed as a user-friendly guide for anyone ready to use essential oils for brain health and looking for a quick and easy way to get started. You may have heard that essential oils are amazing healing tools, but you have no idea where to start. Or, you may already have experience using essential oils and want a simple and easy guide to expand your essential oil knowledge and skills.

You may choose to read the book from beginning to end or read the chapters in any order, based on specific symptoms you might be hoping to address, including sleep, stress, fatigue, brain fog, anxiety, depression, pain, weight gain, immune challenges, or blood sugar challenges. You can also skip ahead to my five-step protocol in Part Two to jump-start your brain health with essential oils.

PART ONE explains the 5 steps and details strategies to help reduce stressors and energy drains on your brain to enhance optimal function.

STEP 1 Shifting the Nervous System into the Parasympathetic Gear

You can activate your body's ability to heal with essential oils by supporting the healthy function of the most important nerve in your body—your vagus nerve. It serves as the on-off switch for many functions in your body, impacting your mood, quality of sleep, digestion, immune function, and, most importantly, your ability to reduce inflammation and heal. Activating the healthy function of your vagus nerve with essential oils amplifies other healing protocols and helps you feel better almost immediately!

STEP 2 Improving Sleep and Detoxifying the Brain

Your brain cleans house while you sleep and helps you reset for the next day. If you are not sleeping, you cannot heal. Once waste washes from the brain, it needs to be eliminated from your body. Using essential oils to remove congestion in your elimination pathways (like your lymphatic system, liver, gallbladder, and gut) ensures that brain waste actually leaves your body and does not recirculate and contribute to brain inflammation and cognitive impairment.

STEP 3 Fueling Your Brain with Energy to Heal

Just like a car, your brain needs fuel to run properly. Brain fuel is oxygen, glucose (or blood sugar), and stimulation. Essential oils can help balance blood sugar and improve circulation. This ensures that your brain receives a healthy supply of glucose (energy), oxygen, and other nutrients it needs to function well and heal quickly. Stimulating blood flow to your brain also helps to improve focus, reduce depression and anxiety, and invoke feelings of calm and control.

STEP 4 Reducing Stress, Improving Mood, and Losing Weight
It takes a lot of energy to heal. Stress patterns hijack all available energy and resources. This depletes your physical and emotional energy, impacting your mood and your waistline. Essential oils can help your brain to shift out of a stress response, freeing up energy and resources that your body can then use to heal, feel happier, and shed extra pounds.

STEP 5 Modulating Your Immune System and Calming Inflammation
Your immune system needs to be working with you, not against you. So often, your immune system is over-reacting (triggering chronic inflammation, food allergies, and autoimmune activity) or under-reacting and setting the stage for chronic illness or brain degeneration. Restoring proper balance of your immune system and calming brain inflammation are critical to healthy brain function. Essential oils, with their antibacterial, antiviral, and antifungal properties, can help reset your immune system and calm an inflammatory response.

PART TWO ties the steps together in a regimen, including the specific sequencing and timing on which oils to use in what order and combination to help turn on your body's full support for healing. Prioritizing health concerns can be a challenge because they often relate to one another. But in my experience, optimal health hinges on the healthy function in the five key areas where your body and brain can fall out of balance.

Nothing in this book is intended to diagnose, treat, or cure any medical conditions or serve as a substitute for professional medical advice. The intention is to empower you to use essential oil blends on specific application points to help balance your organ systems and regions of your brain. General recipes are included for inspiration, but you are also encouraged to create your own blends.

Follow Your Nose

Your sense of smell is the most powerful channel into your body, making inhalation the most direct and effective method of using essential oils, especially for targeting your brain.

Your brain's response to scent triggers nerve impulses that, in turn, stimulate or inhibit the production and release of hormones and neurotransmitters that regulate your bodily functions and alter your emotional response.

Like taste, your brain responds differently to certain types of odor signals. Your brain categorizes odors into two categories: attractive and aversive. Attractive smells activate the release of positive chemical messengers like the bonding hormone oxytocin. Aversive smells activate your fight-or-flight response as well as other important survival functions.

What Happens in Your Brain When You Inhale Essential Oils

When you inhale essential oils, the odor molecules stimulate olfactory receptors in your nasal cavity that then carry the odor information by nerve cells in the form of electrical impulses. In other words, your olfactory receptors transform chemical signals into electrical signals (as opposed to physical signals), which are carried to your olfactory bulb.

Your olfactory bulb, located at the top and on both sides of your inner nasal cavity, is covered with a mucous membrane, known as the olfactory epithelium, which is lined on both sides with about ten million olfactory nerve cells covered with a layer of mucus. Each nerve cell carries a bundle consisting of six to eight tiny hairs, or cilia, equipped with receptor cells. The nerve cells' hairs—up to eighty million of them—are capable of carrying a tremendous amount of information, a capability that outperforms every known analytical human function.

From your olfactory bulb, smell information is routed to other parts of your olfactory system like your olfactory cortex and the limbic area of your brain. Your limbic system serves as the control center in the brain for your emotions and psychological responses like hunger, thirst, and sex drive. This is why scent can influence appetite and sexual attraction.

The cells of the olfactory epithelium are in fact brain cells. This olfactory membrane is the only place in your body where your central nervous system is exposed and is in direct contact with the environment!

How to Inhale Essential Oils

The easiest way to absorb essential oils is literally to smell them. Open the bottle, hold it a few inches below your nose, and inhale deeply. You can also put a drop of oil on your hands, rub them together, and cup your hands over your nose. Another inhalation option includes putting a drop or two on a cotton ball or tissue and placing it in your shirt pocket (or tucking it in under your bra).

Before bedtime, you can also place a few drops of oil on your pillowcase or on a cotton ball near your bed to get a mildly diffused inhalation effect throughout the night. Or you can place a small bowl of Epsom salt on the night table and add 3 to 5 drops of essential oils to the salt. The salt slows the evaporation rate of the oils, so you'll get a longer diffusion throughout the night.

You can also diffuse oils into the air. Diffusing is not as effective or direct as other inhalation or topical application methods for balancing different organs or regions of the brain, but it can be highly effective for neutralizing environmental toxins and mold. When choosing a diffuser, cold diffusion is preferable, since heat can destroy some of the constituents of the oils. If you choose a diffuser that uses heat, ceramic or glass is superior to plastic.

Topical Application

Topical, or transdermal, application allows active ingredients of healing substances to be delivered across the skin. The combination of your skin's permeability to fat-soluble substances and the small size of essential oil molecules make topical application ideal for balancing certain organ systems or stimulating various regions of the brain.

The skin is your largest organ and is relatively permeable to essential oils. For thousands of years, people have placed healing substances on the skin for therapeutic effects. Modern medicine has taken advantage of this transdermal channel, developing a variety of topical formulations to treat local indications. Consider the use of patches for motion sickness, nicotine addiction, contraception, and hormone replacement.

This topical delivery channel is an effective alternative to oral delivery, especially because it bypasses the stomach and liver, both of which can chemically alter the therapeutic effects of drugs and essential oils.

Also, topical application is non-invasive and easy to administer (even for young children or those with serious health or digestive challenges who find other remedies difficult to tolerate or assimilate). For optimal results, you can apply specific blends over the organ systems they are designed to balance. To alleviate anxiety or fatigue, which is often a reflection of underlying adrenal imbalances, you might apply indicated essential oils on the lower back over the adrenal glands.

Applying essential oils to pulse points, like the wrists, the temples, and the back of the neck, where the blood vessels are the closest to the skin, allows for quicker absorption and helps them get to work faster. Absorption can also occur through the hair follicles and sweat ducts or areas of the body with a greater concentration of sweat glands, such as your head and the bottoms of your feet.

Factors that increase the blood flow to the surface of the skin, such as clean skin and pores, the rate of circulation, and the warmth of the skin, also increase the skin's ability to absorb the oils. Activities that increase circulation and warmth, like hot showers, baths, exercise, massage, saunas, or sitting in a warm room will increase the rate of absorption. Similarly, if you massage your skin first, it will increase circulation to that area, thereby causing an increase in absorption of essential oils.

Applying Oils to the Bottoms of the Feet

All oils can be applied to the bottoms of the feet, since the skin there is thicker and less likely to react. The bottoms of the feet contain physical and emotional reflexology points that correspond to energy points or meridians in all of your internal organs, muscular system, skeletal system, and other parts of the body. This connection to internal organs and systems make the bottoms of the feet an effective application point for treating the entire body. If you are sensitive to smell, application on the bottom of the feet can be a good option.

HOW TO APPLY ESSENTIAL OILS TO THE FEET

Reflexology points on the bottoms of the feet correspond to energy points throughout the body.

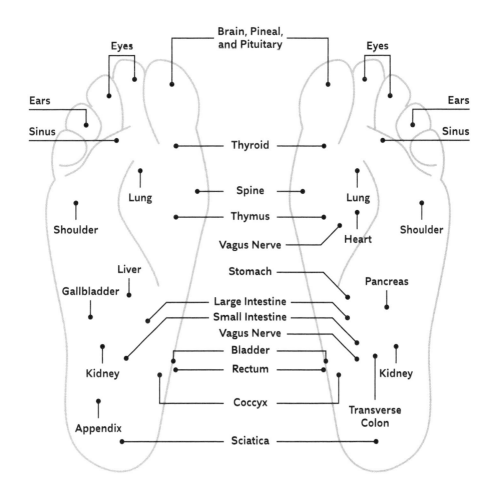

HOW TO APPLY ESSENTIAL OILS TO THE EARS

Reflexology points on the outer ear also correspond to specific organs and emotional states.

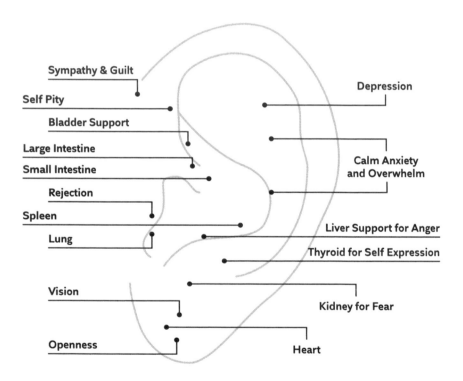

How to Apply Essential Oils to the Ears

Do not place essential oils within your ear canal. The outermost part of the ear contains emotional reflexology points that correspond to specific emotions and meridians of your internal organs. Applying mild pressure to the reflexology points aids in removing emotional and physical blocks and can help restore balance to the body.

In addition to targeting a specific reflex point, you can rub the entire ear to reduce pain, lower blood pressure, balance hormones, and release endorphins into your system. Your earlobes are energetically linked to your brain. When the right earlobe is massaged, it allows the left brain and pituitary gland to become stimulated. When the left earlobe is massaged, it allows the right brain and pineal gland to become stimulated, giving you a whole brain experience. Just use your thumb and index fingers to massage your earlobes gently in small circles. Rubbing your ears with essential oils a few times a day for as little as a minute is an easy way to return your body to balance.

Internal Ingestion

I do not recommend ingesting essential oils. Several studies show that taking essential oils internally is the least effective way to absorb their therapeutic properties. The oil winds up in the digestive tract, where it has to pass through the stomach and the small intestine before it reaches the bloodstream. This process can chemically alter the essential oils and can increase the toxic burden on your liver and kidneys.

I have talked to many people who claim benefits from the internal consumption of essential oils. However, when I dig deeper, I find most of them are adding the oils to water and drinking it. As you drink the water, you inhale the essential oils, so it is likely through the olfactory channel, not the digestive tract, that the oils and their benefits are being assimilated into the body. And it could be that the oils are being absorbed more directly into the bloodstream through the highly sensitive capillaries in the mouth, rather than the digestive tract.

> **Topical Application on Digestive Reflex Points**
>
> In my clinical experience, topical application, especially on digestive reflex points, is equally if not more effective than ingestion. Topical application avoids the hurdles of the digestive process, including exposure to stomach acid and digestive enzymes, and helps prevent elimination via the liver as part of phase I detoxification.

Safety Precautions

Be careful to never apply essential oils in the ear canal, near the eyes, or on an open wound. Oils can be easily absorbed through cuts, scrapes, abrasions, burns, and eczema.

Always test a nickel-sized portion on the inside of the arm or another area of skin to make sure your skin can handle the oil before using. For the first few days of usage, I encourage you to dilute the essential oil with a carrier oil like coconut or olive oil and gradually work up to a recommended dosage.

The viscosity of the carrier oil will impact how easily the oils penetrate the skin. Sweet almond oil and grapeseed oil are less viscous and will penetrate the skin more easily than thicker oils like olive oil, coconut oil, or almond oil.

In the event of any redness or reaction, apply another oil, like coconut oil or olive oil, over the essential oil application to dilute it. Do not use water, as it might further aggravate the reaction.

How Much to Apply? Less Is More

Essential oils are highly concentrated and extremely potent. A drop or two can produce significant results because an entire plant, when distilled, might produce only a single drop of essential oil. Essential oils are approximately 75 to 100 times more concentrated, and consequently far more potent, than dried herbs. For example, 1 drop of peppermint essential oil is considered the therapeutic equivalent to 26 to 28 cups of peppermint tea.

This potency can be used to activate or amplify the healing benefit of foods, supplements, or dried herbs taken in combination with essential oils.

I have long observed that the oils help to activate and enhance the nutrients in the supplements for better absorption and assimilation.

Because they are so concentrated, it is important to ensure that plants used for oils are grown without toxins like pesticides, chemical fertilizers, adulterants, or added synthetic chemicals that would then be concentrated during the distillation process. Look for essential oils that are either certified organic, organically grown in countries that do not offer organic certification, or wildcrafted in nature.

When applying essential oils, less is often more. Smelling the bottle a few inches below the nose for three to seven breaths is often sufficient. In fact, at a certain point, you may find you can no longer smell the blend. This is often an indication that the brain has recognized and transmitted the information of the essential oil molecule. When the sense of smell is satisfied, we often stop detecting the fragrance, since no more is needed at that time. It is a similar mechanism to how we stop eating when our sense of hunger has been satisfied.

Essential oils are very powerful tools for naturally shifting the body into balance and can trigger both a physical and emotional detoxifying response. For that reason, I recommend starting very gradually, first smelling the oil for a few days, then diluting heavily with each topical application to gradually work up to a full dosage. This gradual introduction reduces the chances of an intense reaction.

Like homeopathy, essential oils can be more effective in small amounts. When diffusing, only use the oil to the level of detection (being able to smell it) for short intervals, no more than 20 minutes at a time. Similarly, applying multiple blends at the same time of the day can overstimulate or confuse the body. I advise against applying more than three different blends at any given time during the day.

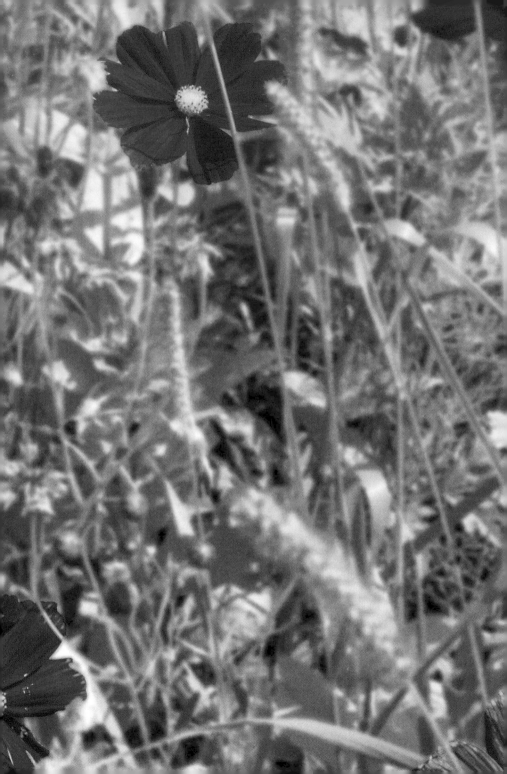

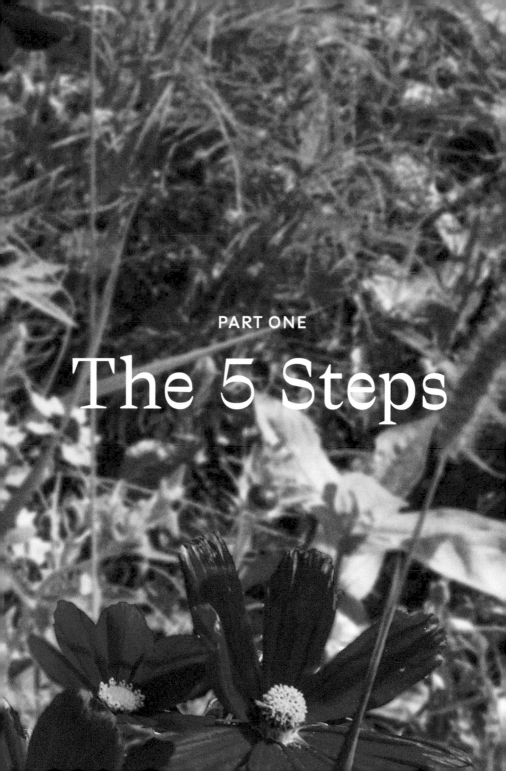

PART ONE

The 5 Steps

SHIFTING THE NERVOUS SYSTEM INTO THE PARASYMPATHETIC GEAR

Repairing the health of your nervous system is the first step in improving your brain function and your physical and emotional health. You simply CANNOT properly address health issues—like gut, immune system, or brain disorders—WITHOUT optimizing vagus nerve function!

The Vagus Nerve and the Parasympathetic State

Your vagus nerve is the primary channel of communication between your brain and your body. Derived from the Latin word *vagus,* which means "wandering," your vagus nerve wanders through the body, connecting your brain with almost every organ. It facilitates two-way communication—carrying messages from your gut, heart, immune system, and other major organs to your brain. In response to these incoming messages, your brain releases the appropriate chemical messengers, like hormones and neurotransmitters, that regulate and control *all* of the unconscious processes in your body, including your heart rate, digestion, appetite, mood, pain threshold, sleep, memory, cognitive function, and immune response.

When your vagus nerve is working optimally, you are likely to recover more quickly after stress, injury, or illness. If your vagus nerve does not properly communicate these signals, or if the signals misfire, your body cannot stay in a state of balance. You may experience feelings of pain, fatigue, brain fog, stress, anxiety, or depression, as well as a number of neurological and even autoimmune issues.

The healthy functioning of your vagus nerve promotes the healthy functioning of the organs, including:

- **brain,** helping to control anxiety and relieve depression.
- **tongue,** helping to improve taste and saliva production, swallowing, and speech.
- **ears,** helping to ease tinnitus.
- **eyes,** helping the pupils shrink to improve focus and make eye contact.
- **stomach,** helping to stimulate stomach acid for healthy digestion.

VAGUS NERVE

Derived from the Latin word *vagus*, which means "wandering," your vagus nerve connects your brain with almost every organ.

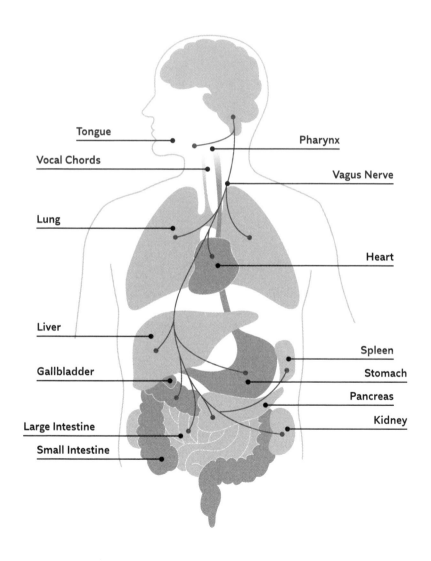

- **intestines,** allowing for nutrient absorption and triggering the muscle contractions to allow food and waste to move through the digestive tract.
- **lungs,** allowing airways to expand and contract.
- **pancreas,** triggering the production and release of enzymes that aid in digestion.
- **liver,** triggering detoxification and supporting blood sugar functions.
- **gallbladder,** triggering the release of bile that rids the body of toxins and breaks down fat (critical for most paleo and keto diets).
- **heart,** helping to control heart rate and blood pressure.
- **spleen,** inhibiting inflammation by calming the release of pro-inflammatory cytokines (substances secreted by inflammatory cells that affect other cells).
- **kidneys,** releasing sodium, increasing blood flow, and managing blood sugar.
- **bladder,** allowing for bladder retention to prevent frequent urination.
- **reproductive organs and genitals,** supporting fertility and sexual arousal.
- **immune system,** regulating inflammation, switching off the production of proteins that fuel the inflammatory immune response.

The Autonomic Nervous System

Just as your car has a gas pedal and brakes, your nervous system has two speeds. The sympathetic fight-or-flight branch automatically helps you accelerate and avoid danger or provides a burst of energy to combat perceived dangers. The parasympathetic rest-digest-and-heal branch slows down the body and shifts it into a response that calms you and allows for recovery and repair after the danger has passed. The gearshift between these two states is your vagus nerve. It facilitates the state of balance between your sympathetic and parasympathetic systems, serving as the on-off switch between the two.

These two-speed states cannot exist at the same time, so when one fires, it inhibits the other. When your vagus nerve activates your parasympathetic rest-and-digest state, it dampens your sympathetic fight-flight-freeze state. The yin and yang pull of these two systems keeps your body in balance. Together they ensure that you have enough resources in the right places at the right time. For example, parasympathetic turns on your digestion, but when you sense danger or feel anxious, your sympathetic branch kicks in and dampens digestion to free up energy for you to mobilize, fight, or flee.

Your autonomic nervous system, which manages all involuntary bodily functions that fall outside of your conscious control—heart rate, blood pressure, digestion, respiration, cell activity, and even body temperature—are built around the balance of these two opposing actions, in rhythmic alternation.

In response to danger, your sympathetic state activates the fight-or-flight response and triggers the release of stress hormones like cortisol and epinephrine (adrenaline) through your body. Your heart rate and blood pressure increase, and digestion slows or stops altogether, as blood is routed away from your internal organs toward your limbs in preparation to fight or flee. Your respiratory rate increases to transport nutrients and oxygen to the cells faster. Your muscles tense, and blood vessels in the extremities constrict. These responses have tremendous value for survival. For example, if you become injured, you are less likely to bleed to death; your pupils dilate so you can see more clearly.

The sympathetic state also down-regulates all functions that are not critical to survival, including all healing and repair processes, like the immune system. A suppressed immune system allows viruses and bacteria to run rampant, contributing to the overgrowth of harmful pathogens in the gut and the potential growth of unhealthy cells such as cancer.

Your parasympathetic nervous system is associated with relaxation, regeneration, and repair. After a danger has passed, your parasympathetic nervous system brings your body back into balance by releasing the neurotransmitter acetylcholine, which helps calm the sympathetic arousal, bringing your heart rate down and helping you relax after periods of stress and anxiety.

All health maintenance processes—including digestion, detoxification, immune activities, tissue regeneration, and arousal—are turned on only when the parasympathetic branch of your nervous system is activated. For simplification purposes, I refer to this as the "parasympathetic state." The parasympathetic state activates your ability to heal. It brings your nervous system into balance and affects EVERY aspect of your well-being! Simply put: you cannot heal outside of the parasympathetic state.

You should optimally be in a parasympathetic state 80 percent of the time, but many people struggle to be in this state at any point during their day. Almost all disease and dysfunction result from not being able to drop into the parasympathetic state.

Parasympathetic Quiz

Test yourself: Does this sound like you? If so, then you may need help shifting into the parasympathetic state.

——— Dry mouth or eyes
——— Clenched or grinding teeth
——— Lump in your throat or difficulty swallowing
——— Acid reflux
——— Bloating or burping after fatty or fried meals
——— Poor digestion (bloating, gas, slow food motility)
——— Slow bowel movements or a tendency for constipation
——— Digestive disorders, including a leaky gut and food allergies, irritable bowel syndrome (IBS), small intestine bacterial overgrowth (SIBO), or Crohn's disease
——— Floating stools
——— Not being able to tell when you are full or hungry
——— Frequent urination or incontinence
——— Difficulty relaxing
——— Tendency for anxiety
——— Episodes of a racing heart
——— Tense muscles, especially around the neck or shoulder
——— Sleep problems, insomnia, or nightmares
——— Low libido or erectile dysfunction
——— Cognitive dysfunction, ADHD, or autism
——— Brain fog
——— Easily startled
——— Chronic inflammation or infections
——— Sensitive to bright or flashing lights
——— Migraines, dizziness, tinnitus, or vertigo
——— High or low blood pressure
——— Tendency for depression
——— Vitamin B$_{12}$ deficiency
——— Low vitamin D or other nutrient levels

The Benefits of a Functioning Parasympathetic System

Once you stimulate the vagus nerve with essential oils to shift into the parasympathetic state, your body shifts into balance, improving many functions from digestion to cognition.

IMPROVES DIGESTION

How you eat may be more important than what you eat, because proper digestion occurs only in a parasympathetic state. You need to invest not only in a pristine diet but also in taking the time to eat in a calm, relaxed atmosphere to get the most nutrients from food and ensure that nutrients are properly delivered to your cells. If you eat under stress, the nutrients in your food will not be properly digested, absorbed, or assimilated. Think of an ambulance that is stuck in traffic and can't make it to the person in need. That is what is happening in our bodies when we eat under stress: nutrients aren't making it into the cells to help us heal.

When you eat in the parasympathetic state, the brain activates all of your digestive functions, including the production of saliva and the release of stomach acid, enzymes, and bile. This supports nutrient assimilation and motility, also called peristalsis, or the muscle contractions required to move food and waste through your system. The parasympathetic state allows the gut to signal the brain about hunger and satiety, helping you recognize when you are truly hungry or full.

Finally, if your stomach doesn't release acid and enzymes to break down proteins, these undigested proteins can trigger an immune response. Adding essential oils to stimulate your parasympathetic response before meals helps your body better absorb nutrients, which, in turn, helps to heal many of the following digestive disorders.

> **SIBO.** Peristalsis is a wavelike motion in the gut that moves food, mucus, bacteria, and fungi along the digestive tract. This "housekeeping wave" normalizes mobility to resolve SIBO.
>
> **IBS.** Poor communication between the gut and the brain may cause abdominal pain, constipation, and/or diarrhea (symptoms of IBS). The parasympathetic state improves signals between the gut and brain.
>
> **Constipation.** Peristalsis, the muscle contractions of the intestines that move the stool, is triggered by the parasympathetic state.
>
> **Acid indigestion or gastroesophageal reflux disease (GERD).** The parasympathetic state signals the sphincter between your stomach and esophagus to close, preventing acid reflux from stomach to esophagus.

Bloating. Bloating is an indication of a stomach acid or enzyme deficiency. The parasympathetic state supports the body's production of adequate acid and enzymes for digestion.

Bile stasis. The parasympathetic state triggers bile production and signals the gallbladder to release bile into the intestines to digest dietary fats.

Dry mouth. The parasympathetic state initiates the production of saliva, which is critical to good periodontal health and digestion.

Anorexia and bulimia. The parasympathetic state allows the gut to send to the brain signals of hunger and satiety.

SPEEDS DETOXIFICATION

Your body's mechanism of eliminating toxins only occurs in the parasympathetic state. The vagus nerve, which triggers the parasympathetic response, connects to all the organs of detoxification including the lungs, spleen, kidney, small intestine, liver, gallbladder, stomach, and colon. Triggering the parasympathetic state with essential oils helps route blood flow to these organs to enhance detoxification.

COMBATS INFLAMMATION

The parasympathetic state reduces inflammation in your body and brain. Your vagus nerve helps detect and calm inflammation, alerting your brain to release the anti-inflammatory neurotransmitter acetylcholine, which acts as a brake on inflammation in your body. When your vagus nerve isn't functioning properly, these anti-inflammatory signals are not sent, setting the stage for chronic inflammatory issues.

BOOSTS IMMUNITY

The parasympathetic state turns on your immune processes, allowing your body to fight:

——— *Helicobacter pylori*, intestinal bacteria that contribute to acid reflux and stomach ulcers
——— Candida or yeast infections
——— Fungal infections
——— Periodontal infections (saliva production protects the mouth from infections)
——— Chronic sinus, respiratory, gut, or urinary infections

REDUCES SYMPTOMS OF DEPRESSION

Stimulating your vagus nerve with essential oils "can significantly reduce multiple symptoms of depression, including anxiety, sleep disturbance, and hopelessness," according to a study in *Frontiers in Psychiatry*. A growing body of research suggests that stress and inflammation initiate mental and physical processes that increase the risk for depression. In contrast, activating the parasympathetic state reduces inflammation and improves connectivity in brain regions involved in depression and mood regulation. Citrus essential oils, like lime, were found to be effective at combating depression in a study called "Effects of Citrus Fragrance on Immune Function and Depressive States," by scientists in the journal *Neuroimmunomodulation*.

DECREASES ANXIETY

Anxiety is a repetitive experience of fear that occurs when fight-or-flight survival mechanisms are activated. When your fear response is fired up, everything else needs to shut down to devote your body's metabolism and energy to stay alert to potential or imminent danger. The sympathetic fight-or-flight branch of your nervous system controls anxiety, readying your muscles to flee, increasing your heart and respiratory rate, increasing your blood pressure, and motivating you to do something. This is why anxiety promotes twitches, shaking legs, twirling of hair, and pacing. It says move, act, fight, or flee. In contrast, the parasympathetic state promotes the feeling of safety—slowing your heart rate and normalizing rapid breathing—to help shift you out of anxiety.

RELIEVES PAIN

The parasympathetic state can help reduce pain perception. Pain is a signal from your brain to your body. When you calm your brain by helping it drop into the parasympathetic state, you help calm your pain. Research by doctors published in *Pain Practice*, the official journal of the World Institute of Pain, on high-anxiety subjects has found that their pain perception dropped significantly when they were in the parasympathetic state. Extreme athletes also recover more quickly from exercise when they activate the parasympathetic state.

Clove oil has been used for centuries to help treat and relieve pain. Clove oil's anti-inflammatory, antispasmodic, and analgesic properties make it an ideal natural painkiller. It is thought to work by blocking nerve signals from sending the message of pain from the body to the brain, thus giving the user a break from pain. The warming characteristic of clove oil is thought to provide numbing relief from pain, and the antioxidants found in this oil assist in the protection of cells.

IMPROVES GUT HEALTH

Your vagus nerve is the link between your gut and your brain. Ninety percent of the nerve fibers in your gut connect to your brain via your vagus nerve.

Your gut is the largest sampling site for what exists in your environment. Everything that enters your body—through your mouth, nose, eyes, and even your ears—drains into your digestive track. Gut microbes communicate through the vagus nerve to trigger an immune response in your brain, heart, lungs, and skeletal muscles. The parasympathetic state helps keep this gut flora healthy by sending increased blood flow to the gut, which supports healthy motility, enzyme secretion, and nutrient absorption while activating the beneficial effects of the probiotic bacteria.

CALMS STRESS

The first line of defense against stress is the fight-or-flight survival response triggered by the sympathetic nervous system. This activates stress symptoms like a racing heartbeat, increased blood pressure, and respiratory rate, as blood flow is routed toward the muscles in the arms and legs in preparation for flight. Activating the parasympathetic state signals that the danger has passed and allows you to rest and recover.

INCREASES ADRENAL HEALTH

Although your autonomic nervous system does not directly control the adrenals, a chronic sympathetic fight-or-flight response can trigger your adrenal glands to produce high amounts of the stress hormone cortisol, which can push the body into adrenal fatigue. The parasympathetic state normalizes this stress response, helping to put the brakes on excessive cortisol output, which can help heal the adrenals.

BOOSTS ENERGY

Your body and brain need energy and vitality to heal. Energy fuels your body's internal functions and repairs, building and maintaining cells and tissues and facilitating the chemical reactions that allow you to heal. When you are stuck in the sympathetic fight-or-flight state, your ability to regenerate, digest, detoxify, and heal slows down dramatically, allowing toxins to accumulate, contributing to your sense of fatigue. When you help your body drop into the healing parasympathetic state, it can finally get rid of the accumulated toxins and start to regain energy and vitality. Your mind and body can also relax, which slows the release of cortisol and allows for optimal energy flow.

IMPROVES HEART HEALTH

Your heart rate is controlled by a delicate balance between the two states of your nervous system. The fight-or-flight sympathetic nervous system raises your heart rate to pump more blood to the muscles and flee from danger, whereas the rest-and-digest parasympathetic nervous system slows down the heart rate so you can recover. The vagus nerve serves as a temperate gauge to control your heart rate via electrical impulses to specialized muscle tissue—the heart's natural pacemaker—in the right atrium. The vagus nerve releases the neurotransmitter acetylcholine, which prolongs the time between heartbeats, thus slowing your pulse.

Heart health requires daily regeneration of the heart, and we regenerate in the parasympathetic state. Research links heart disease with increased sympathetic activity.

INCREASES MUSCLE STRENGTH

Your vagus nerve releases acetylcholine, which controls the communication between your nerves and your muscles, causing your muscles to contract so you can move. Low levels of acetylcholine may contribute to muscle weakness or fatigue that worsens with exercise or exertion. The muscles may work for a while, but ultimately they exhaust their supply of acetylcholine, leading to extreme fatigue.

ENHANCES SEXUAL HEALTH

Sexual arousal is a parasympathetic event. The vagus nerve connects to your genital organs to increase blood flow and sensation. The vagus nerve innervates the female cervix and the uterus and is one of the major nerve pathways that transmit sexual and orgasmic energy signals from the genitals to the brain. Erectile dysfunction is often associated with insufficient blood flow to the genitals, so stimulating the parasympathetic response can increase blood flow to the area.

BALANCES BLOOD SUGAR

Stress increases blood sugar and insulin output. Research with mice showed a correlation between a significant drop in blood sugar levels following the stimulation of the parasympathetic nervous system. Your sympathetic nervous system is activated in response to falling blood sugar. As the body perceives this as an emergency, the parasympathetic state can be triggered to balance blood sugar levels.

ALLEVIATES TRAUMA AND POST-TRAUMATIC STRESS DISORDER (PTSD)

Trauma often occurs when perceived danger tips your nervous system into the "fight-flight-or-freeze" survival mode. When that trauma is not processed, your nervous system can get stuck in that survival mode and replay the experience of the initial trauma, even in safe surroundings. To heal trauma, you must shift your nervous system out of survival mode and toward the parasympathetic "safe" state.

RELIEVES INSOMNIA

Access to a parasympathetic state allows for relaxation, helps quiet brain chatter, and allows for deeper levels of sleep. When the sympathetic nervous system is overactive, the body gets stuck in a chronic stress response. In this state, increased levels of the stress hormone cortisol are produced, which stimulates the mind and body to a highly alert and wakeful state. High cortisol levels also depress the sleep hormone melatonin. Activating the parasympathetic nervous system allows the body to relax and release melatonin, which enhances your ability to sleep.

REGULATES APPETITE AND WEIGHT

Your vagus nerve controls communication between your gut and your brain, including messages of hunger and satiety that are best communicated in the parasympathetic state. Poor communication leads to over- or under-eating and can contribute to eating disorders like anorexia and bulimia. When your vagus nerve stimulates the parasympathetic state and is able to clearly communicate signals of hunger or fullness to your brain, you feel appropriately hungry or satiated and are then able to achieve healthy body weight.

Research from the University of California San Diego School of Medicine has found that individuals suffering from anorexia nervosa respond differently to hunger signals, noting that "brain circuitry differences in anorexics make them less sensitive to reward and the motivational drive of hunger." Supporting the parasympathetic state and optimal vagus nerve function helps improve brain mechanisms that support appetite regulation.

STRENGTHENS MEMORY

Emotionally arousing or meaningful events generate strong memories to foster sentimental pleasure and help avoid future danger. Stimulating the vagus nerve can strengthen memory. When the vagus nerve is stimulated, it triggers

Essential oils help bring energy to specific organ systems and cells to temporarily stimulate or increase the activity of the organ system. For example, topically applied essential oils can help stimulate your vagus nerve and reboot your system, manually overriding impaired function and resetting the autonomic nervous system. The fat-soluble essential oils are able to pass through your skin to directly and immediately access your vagus nerve in a way that other supplements or remedies cannot.

the release of the neurotransmitter norepinephrine into an area of the brain called the amygdala, which strengthens memory storage and improves your ability to process and retain information.

ENHANCES BREATHING

Your vagus nerve tells your lungs when it is time to breathe and communicates with your diaphragm to produce deep breaths. Deep, calming diaphragm breathing plays a key role in healing practices like yoga and meditation, all of which activate the parasympathetic state.

Vagus Nerve Dysfunction

Any damage or congestion in your vagus nerve can both compromise communication between the brain and the organs and impede drainage of toxins from the brain. Such damage or congestion will simultaneously affect all downstream functions of various systems in your body. This dysfunction, which is also called toxicity, may be the most common undiagnosed issue with chronic illness. Clinicians such as chronic disease specialist Dr. Dietrich Klinghardt finds compromised vagus nerve function in more than 95 percent of his chronically ill patients.

Harvard researcher and clinician Dr. Datis Kharrazian shares similar findings in his book *Why Isn't My Brain Working?* He notes that 90 percent of the brain's output goes through the brain stem, and healthy brain function generates a parasympathetic response, while at the same time dampening the sympathetic system. Kharrazian finds that when brain regions start slowing down and losing function, there is less output into the part of the brain stem that triggers parasympathetic activity, leading to an increase in sympathetic activity. To put it more simply, a poorly functioning brain does not stimulate the vagus nerve.

The health of your vagus nerve is of utmost importance to the health of your brain, immune system, and the body's ability to fight inflammation. Since your vagus nerve is the primary information highway between your body and your brain, any congestion impedes communication. Your brain functions best when messages get delivered quickly and clearly. Compromised vagus nerve function diminishes the strength and speed of these signals. Messages are not properly delivered or received. Organs cannot get what they need from your brain, and your brain cannot get what it needs from your organs, contributing to symptoms like fatigue, brain fog, and physical pain.

Vagus nerve toxicity can be an underlying root cause for many chronic diseases, including autoimmune diseases, fibromyalgia, chronic fatigue syndrome, postural orthostatic tachycardia syndrome (POTS), depression, anxiety, bipolar disorder, digestive disorders like SIBO and IBS, diabetes, heart disease, and even obesity.

How Toxicity Impedes Health

Vagus nerve toxicity is one way these signals can be compromised. Toxicity alters the production of neurotransmitters, such as GABA (gamma-aminobutyric acid), which can reduce anxiety, improve your mood, and affect other hormones that impact your brain function and mental health.

SYMPTOMS OF VAGUS NERVE TOXICITY

Since your vagus nerve connects your brain to all of your major organ systems, any interference in its ability to send signals back and forth can affect virtually every part of your body. As a result, you may experience any of the following:

- Anxiety
- Depression
- Chronic fatigue
- Forgetfulness and brain fog
- Autoimmune conditions
- Digestive challenges, including small intestine bacterial overgrowth (SIBO), irritable bowel syndrome (IBS), acid reflux, and Crohn's disease
- Systemic inflammation and leaky gut
- Migraines
- Fibromyalgia or chronic pain
- Insomnia

- Tinnitus
- Thyroid disorders
- Loss of appetite
- Weight gain
- Heart problems
- Nausea or dizziness
- Heartburn
- Blood sugar imbalances
- Constant thirst
- Frequent urination
- Unexplained ear or neck pain
- Chest pressure
- Shortness of breath
- Cold or heat sensitivity (especially in hands or feet)
- Fuzzy thoughts and words
- Panic attacks
- Feelings of being overwhelmed
- Decreased muscle strength

What Causes Vagus Nerve Toxicity?

Poor health can often be traced to a vagus nerve poisoned by neurotoxins. Toxins that affect your brain and nervous system are lipophilic (fat loving) and easily absorbed by nerve endings. They can disrupt critical functions of your cells, including the transport of nutrients and oxygen. These toxins include heavy metals; antibiotics; bacteria, viruses, and parasites; biotoxins; and environmental toxins. Toxins drain from the brain down the lymph channels on the sides of the neck. If lymph flow in the neck is congested, toxins can build up and linger, affecting the vagus nerve and preventing cellular waste from exiting the brain.

For example, toxins present in the mouth (including bacteria from infected root canals or cavitations in the jawbone), tonsils, and sinuses also drain into the lymph system in your neck via your trigeminal nerve (along your jawbone), where it intersects with your vagus nerve on the side of the neck. You might think of your neck as a crowded multilane highway with a lot of traffic. Congestion can block movement, causing toxins to linger and damage the vagus nerve.

HEAVY METALS

Heavy metals, like mercury, aluminum, lead, and cadmium, have a high affinity for nerves. Your nerve endings absorb metals, which then travel through your nerves, including your vagus nerve, toward your brain stem, where they can impact other brain tissues.

Because of the immense networking of nerves, toxins can be quickly absorbed in massive amounts, disrupting vital functions of your nerve cells. What's more, large concentrations of heavy metals reduce the effectiveness of immune cells, depriving them of blood, nutrients, and oxygen. These areas become havens for anaerobic bacteria, fungi, and viruses, contributing to disease.

Over the last five hundred years, the amount of toxic metals found in human bodies has increased a thousandfold. Heavy metals can be found in food, air, water, personal-care products, and in your teeth if you have amalgam fillings (which are 49.5 percent mercury).

The presence of mercury in the system has an amplifying effect, increasing the toxicity and the damage of other neurotoxins. When mercury is removed, the body starts to effectively eliminate all other neurotoxins.

Health experts believe the presence of heavy metals may cause an overgrowth of yeast or candida, which binds to heavy metals and thus prevents them from entering the bloodstream, shielding and protecting the body from the toxicity of metals. When metals are removed, candida overgrowth is often eliminated.

Heavy metal toxicity can lead to symptoms like headaches, tinnitus, neuropathy, cognitive dysfunction, sleep disorders, constipation, kidney failure, hypertension, muscle weakness, light sensitivity, depression, anxiety, impaired fertility, and anemia.

ANTIBIOTICS

A class of antibiotics known as fluoroquinolones, used to treat a variety of digestive, respiratory, and urinary tract ailments, has been linked with nerve damage since 2004. Fluoroquinolones are marketed as prescription medications, including ciprofloxacin (Cipro), gemifloxacin (Factive), levofloxacin (Levaquin), moxifloxacin (Avelox), norfloxacin (Noroxin), and ofloxacin (Floxin).

These antibiotics can damage your vagus nerve, along with other nerves that send information to and from the brain. They can interrupt the connection between your brain and your body and result in symptoms that include numbness, tingling, burning, or shooting pain.

BACTERIA, VIRUSES, AND PARASITES

Your vagus nerve can become infected with bacteria, like *Borrelia* that cause Lyme disease, viruses such as Epstein-Barr virus (EBV), or parasites. In his vagus nerve infection hypothesis, Tufts University neuroscientist Dr. Michael VanElzakker proposes that nerve-loving microbes in or around the vagus nerve trigger an ongoing immune response that either blocks communication (signaling between cells) or sends alarm signals between cells and tissues.

Blocked communication and miscommunication inhibit the healthy allocation of energy and resources to your body and brain. This triggers symptoms like ongoing and intense pain, fatigue, depression, and a hyper-sensitivity to chemicals, setting the stage for chronic illness.

Because your vagus nerve serves as your immune system's conduit to the brain, VanElzakker believes that even a minor infection in the vagus nerve can wreak havoc in the brain. For example, a biological trigger (like a tick bite) or psychological stress can weaken your immune system, allowing latent opportunistic viruses such as EBV and herpes to become activated (which helps explain how stress triggers disease).

Once activated, these viruses quickly replicate and move upstream inside the nerves toward the brain, where they turn on immune cells in the brain (known as glial cells). This triggers a vicious immune cycle, where brain immune cells release pro-inflammatory chemicals in response to a virus or infection, signaling your vagus nerve to shift your body into "sickness response," where pain, fatigue, brain fog, and flulike symptoms force you to stop moving, eating, and thinking, so that energy can be focused on healing.

In other words, an infection in your vagus nerve can flip a switch in your immune system that keeps you stuck in this exaggerated sickness response, causing ongoing increased sensitivity to pain, fatigue, and chemicals. At its most extreme, the nervous system can interpret even the slightest touch as a signal to induce pain.

ENVIRONMENTAL TOXINS AND BIOTOXINS LIKE MOLD

Toxins drain down the lymph channels along the sides of your neck that run parallel to your vagus nerve. Airborne toxins, such as mold or their mycotoxin by-product and off-gassing chemicals such as wood preservatives and formaldehyde from furniture, and volatile organic compounds (VOCs) from paint drain from your sinuses. Ingested toxins such as pesticides, herbicides, food preservatives, aspartame, and food colorings drain from your mouth, overloading and congesting lymph circulation in the neck. Molecular biologist and radiology specialist Dr. Marco Ruggiero has studied how congested and inflamed lymph vessels compress the vagus nerve and compromise its function, using diagnostic ultrasounds on the neck. He found that mold triggers a chronic inflammatory response that likely congests lymph vessels and compresses the vagus nerve.

OTHER CAUSES OF TOXICITY OR DYSFUNCTION

The vagus nerve can also be affected by psychological and physical experiences including early childhood abuse, neglect, and trauma. The Adverse Childhood Experiences (ACE) questionnaire, created by Kaiser Permanente and the Centers for Disease Control and Prevention, found that trauma and stress early in life—such as family dysfunction like divorce, domestic violence, incarceration, and alcohol and drug issues—triggered a pattern of over-activation of the vagus nerve stress response that correlates with a higher risk of developing chronic health problems in adulthood as well as emotional and social issues such as depression, domestic violence, and suicide.

Stress

Stress triggers your vagus nerve to activate the sympathetic "survival" state of your nervous system. Your heart beats faster, pumping blood to your extremities; your respiratory rate increases; and your pupils dilate to help you hyper-focus and stay alive. After the danger has passed, your body then drops back into a balanced parasympathetic rest-and-digest state, where you can rest, recover, and repair.

Chronic or prolonged periods of stress keep you stuck in the sympathetic state and compromise your vagal tone, or the ability of your vagus nerve to toggle between the parasympathetic and sympathetic states. This can take a toll on your long-term health. The hormones that are released during the stress response, like cortisol, can damage your body, contributing to systemic inflammation and inhibiting your body's immune response.

Physical Trauma

The vagus nerve is such a long nerve, affecting so many areas, and it can be physically damaged at multiple points. Any kind of physical trauma can put pressure on your vagus nerve and irritate it. Serious trauma can occur during surgery if the vagus nerve is cut. But even mild compression of the vagus nerve from whiplash, poor posture, or muscular imbalances may cause it to misfire, leading to overstimulation or desensitization of the nerve.

Emotional Trauma

Emotional trauma—including grief, loss, accidents, any exposure to natural disasters, or verbal and physical violence—can also impact your vagus nerve. During times of heightened stress, your vagus nerve signals your brain to rapidly store memories that are important for your survival. Your subconscious mind doesn't distinguish memories from worries about the future. Similarly, your body cannot differentiate actual physical stress from emotional or antici-patory stress, like trauma or the mental replay of survival-based memories that attempt to predict potential stressors that could occur in some imaginary future. This is common in post–traumatic stress disorder (PTSD).

In the book *Why Zebras Don't Get Ulcers,* Robert M. Sapolsky talks about this phenomenon, noting that "sometimes we are smart enough to see things coming and, based only on anticipation, can turn on a stress response as robust as if the event had actually occurred. Thus, the stress response can be mobilized not only in response to physical or psychological insults, but also in expectation of them." This trauma loop can cause the vagus nerve to freeze, immobilizing you in a kind of suspended animation in response to life-threatening situations and keeping the nerve stuck in that state. For example, if a survivor of gun violence hears a car backfire, they might assume it is the sound of gunshots and remain frozen and paralyzed. The ability to move out of that frozen state and activate optimal vagus nerve function is an important step in reclaiming emotional health for PTSD victims.

If you are experiencing PTSD, any stimulus can activate the frozen trauma response rather than the appropriate orienting reflex (the immediate response to a change in environment), when that change is not sudden enough to elicit the startle reflex.

Trauma can also contribute to vagus nerve toxicity, shifting you into the freeze response. Stress prompts your body to assess, prioritize, and support the following survival options.

Fight. If you assess a danger as something you potentially have the power to defeat, your body drops into a "fight" mode. Your sympathetic nervous system releases hormones like adrenaline that prime you for battle.

Flight. If the danger is too powerful to overcome, your body prepares you to flee. Your system shifts resources and blood flow to your muscles and limbs and shuts down all functions not critical to your immediate survival (like digestion, detoxification, immune function, reproduction, and rational thinking) so you can harness all available energy to escape the danger at hand.

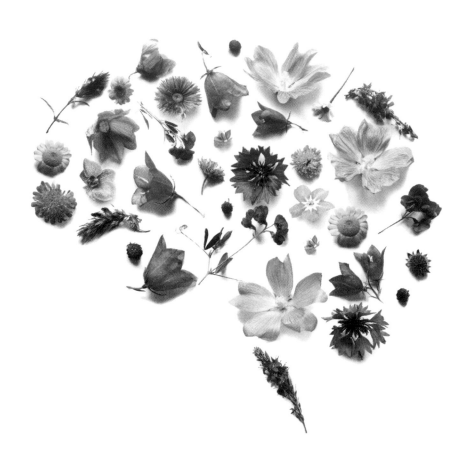

Freeze. If you can neither defeat the dangerous opponent nor safely flee from it, your body drops into a self-paralyzing freeze response. You may be temporarily unable to move, or you may "space out," "freeze up," become numb, or feel as if you had left your body. Your body does not release the hormones to help you fight or flee. It releases chemicals that help dull the pain and numb the intensity of any mental, physical, or emotional injury. This allows you to move through the enormity of what is happening to you and survive the trauma. If you can't make a dangerous individual or situation disappear, you're much better off "disappearing" yourself, by blocking out what's much too scary to take in. For example, a freeze response is often activated in response to child abuse. Childhood distress often correlates with adverse health problems in later life, as measured by the ACE assessments. It is believed that early trauma can keep children stuck in the freeze response and damage vagus nerve function, negatively impacting health throughout their lifetimes.

The freeze state does not allow you to naturally discharge this energy, and that trapped energy, along with the corresponding thoughts and emotions of fear or panic, can stay trapped in your body. It keeps your brain and nervous system in a perpetual state of high alert, damaging your vagus nerve.

All three of these states—fight, flight, and freeze—require your nervous system to shift into a highly energized state. The acts of fighting and fleeing allow your nervous system to discharge this heightened energy and move back into a state of normal function.

In nature, animals often shake or experience rhythmic waves of muscle contractions when they come out of a freeze response. Humans often override or avoid the trembling or shaking that would help drain off the energy of the freeze response, keeping the sympathetic nervous system activated. When your body is stuck in the freeze response, it can provoke paralyzing symptoms like panic attacks, obsessive-compulsive behaviors, avoidance behaviors, phobias, spaciness, numbing out, and other anxiety states.

A healthy vagus nerve lets you know you are safe and that you can relax and heal. When you are stuck in a trauma loop or freeze response, you feel under attack and nothing feels safe to you, including your loved ones. You are unable to connect to others when your freeze mechanism is in high gear.

When my kids were little, one of their preschool teachers suggested that we "connect before we correct," meaning that when they had misbehaved, it was best not to discipline them in the heat of the moment when stuck in the fight-flight-or-freeze state but rather to connect to them through physical touch or gentle words. This connection fostered a sense of safety so that my children could move out of the freeze and fear state and into a more receptive parasympathetic state, where they were able to properly receive my feedback.

When your body is in a state of emergency, it shuts down all functions not relevant to immediate survival, including your ability to connect to others. You can see when another person is in this emergency sympathetic state, unable to connect, by the size of their pupils. When you are under stress, your sympathetic nervous system stimulates your pupils to dilate (making the black circle larger), which lets in more light and improves your vision and ability to focus to enhance your chances for survival. It also prevents you from any visual distraction that may divert your safety-oriented focus. When you feel safe again, your pupils will constrict (making the black circle smaller). Assessing pupil size and the ability to make eye contact is a great way to tell how safe the people in your life are feeling and how open they are to connecting in that moment. For example, if someone you love has dilated pupils, you might wait to bring up a controversial topic until you see the pupil size shrink. This is one reason why eye contact is so important in increasing feelings of connection as well as in healing your vagus nerve.

Smelling Essential Oils Can Thaw the Freeze Response

The freeze response can trigger disassociation so that you don't feel pain. It can also cause you to lose connection to your five senses, including your sense of smell. The sense of smell and essential oils help thaw the freeze response and restore your ability to sense your environment.

Calming your nervous system with essential oils, especially calming citrus oils like orange and bergamot, can help you be present in your body and in the moment. This sense of embodiment and safety can prevent future freeze responses. Taking it one step further by stimulating your vagus nerve with essential oils helps discharge excess energy, shift out of the freeze state, and heal your vagus nerve.

Vagus Nerve Stimulation

My old corporation had a use it or lose it policy when it came to accrued vacation time. Your vagus nerve works in a similar fashion. If you don't use it and develop what is known as vagal tone—the resilience to toggle between the parasympathetic and sympathetic nervous system actions—it doesn't work as well. It could even atrophy. You might think of it like muscle tone. If you don't use your muscle, it atrophies. Stress, toxins, and trauma keep your vagal switch stuck in the off mode.

A key strategy for toning your vagus nerve is to stimulate it. Stimulation activates communication between your body and your brain that triggers the release of different chemical messengers, like neurotransmitters, which improve communication between all the organ systems connected to your vagus nerve.

Vagus Nerve Stimulation Devices

Your vagus nerve travels down your neck near the carotid artery and jugular vein. Neurologists in the nineteenth century noticed that applying pressure on the carotid artery in the neck could stop seizures. This prompted significant research trials, resulting in the development of a battery-powered device, similar to a pacemaker, that is surgically implanted under the skin to stimulate the vagus nerve.

An incision is made on the left side of the neck, and a thin wire is threaded under the skin, connecting the device to the vagus nerve. When activated, the device sends electrical signals along the vagus nerve to the brain stem, which then sends signals to certain areas of the brain. This electrical vagus nerve stimulation has been used to treat epilepsy, depression, multiple sclerosis, migraines, and Alzheimer's disease. The Food and Drug Administration officially approved vagus nerve stimulation for epilepsy in 1997 and for depression in 2005.

Vagus Nerve Stimulation for Inflammation

In 2012, New York neurosurgeon Kevin Tracey found that vagus nerve stimulation devices significantly reduced systemic inflammation and the pain associated with arthritis. The research revealed that inflammation in body tissues was directly regulated by the brain with the vagus nerve serving as the on-off switch—what Tracey coined as the "inflammatory reflex." When the vagus nerve was stimulated, it reduced inflammation elsewhere in the body, by calming the production of the pro-inflammatory chemical messengers.

Other researchers are now looking into using vagus nerve stimulation for other inflammatory conditions like ADD and ADHD, asthma, eczema, anxiety, diabetes, headaches, fatigue, pain, gas, bloating, IBS (irritable bowel syndrome), mood swings, brain fog, and autoimmunity.

Vagal Tone

When you stimulate your vagus nerve, you improve resilience, meaning that your vagus nerve is healthier and more responsive. This allows your body to recover faster after a stressful experience. This measure of balance and resilience in your vagus nerve is referred to as vagal tone.

Strong vagal tone means that signals from your brain and body are better received, allowing you to relax and recover more quickly. This state correlates with greater resilience to stress, shorter recovery times, and better mental and emotional health, including better concentration, memory, and mood. A strong vagal tone enables your body to better regulate blood glucose levels, calm inflammation, and prevent brain degeneration.

Low vagal tone means this regulation is less effective—there is less balance and less resilience—and this can lead to excessive inflammation and disease.

HOW IS VAGAL TONE MEASURED?

Vagal tone is measured through changes in heart rate that occur with the breath, called heart rate variability (HRV). Healthy vagal tone involves a slight increase in heart rate when you inhale and a decrease in heart rate when you exhale. Breathing and meditation techniques work on the principle of improving HRV.

Every time you breathe in, your heart beats faster to speed the flow of oxygenated blood around your body. When you breathe out, your heart rate slows down. A device, called an electrocardiogram, can be used to measure the difference in your heart rate between your inhalation and exhalation to reveal your level of vagal tone. The bigger the difference between your inhalation heart rate and your exhalation heart rate, the stronger your vagal tone.

The Use of Essential Oils for Stimulation

While I discourage applying essential oils directly in the ear canal, topically applying stimulatory essential oils behind the earlobe on the mastoid bone is an incredibly easy, natural, non-invasive remedy for accessing and stimulating the vagus nerve.

In his book *Activate Your Vagus Nerve,* Dr. Navaz Habib details how the skin around your ear can be stimulated to allow optimal signaling to your body and brain. This is the most accessible point on the skin to stimulate your vagus nerve.

Essential oils have both olfactory (smell) and transdermal (topical application) qualities. For example, inhaling essential oils such as lavender or bergamot has been shown to improve HRV, indicating the strengthening of vagal tone. What's more, topically applied essential oils can cross the blood-brain barrier to stimulate communication of the vagus nerve and improve cognition.

You can also activate any of the parts of the body that are enervated by the vagus nerve, including your throat, facial muscles, heart, lungs, and gallbladder. Any practices that stimulate the actions of these areas of the body can influence the functioning of the vagus nerve through the mind-body feedback loop. For example, the vagus nerve runs through the diaphragm and is stimulated with every inhale and exhale.

NOT ALL TOPICAL APPLICATION POINTS ARE CREATED EQUAL

Different application points yield different results. You can significantly amplify your results by intentionally applying essential oils on specific healing points, known as acupuncture points or reflexology points, that are correlated with specific organ systems or regions of the brain. Acupuncture points behind the ear and around the neck are the most effective points for stimulating the vagus nerve. A neural anatomy study on acupuncture points showed the vagus nerve is most accessible for stimulation via the lower half of the back of the ear.

Research on acupuncture and vagus nerve stimulation (VNS) has found that acupuncture points produce clinical benefits through the stimulation of the vagus nerve and/or its branches in the head and neck region that are anatomically proximate to vagus nerve pathways, where the VNS electrode is surgically implanted.

Combining Essential Oils with Acupuncture

Essential oils stimulate acupuncture points and can be as electromagnetically powerful as acupuncture needles, according to Peter Holmes, co-founder of Aroma Acupoint Therapy. Holmes applies essential oil on specific acupuncture points instead of stimulating them with a needle and has found that while both essential oils and needles stimulated the points in a similar way, essential oils also enhance the energy of those points.

The application of specific essential oils on targeted acupuncture points amplifies the benefit of both, achieving a greater therapeutic effect than either remedy in isolation. What's more, stimulating the vagus nerve reflex point helps mimic the energetic signals that the vagus nerve emits to communicate rapidly with other parts of the body and brain.

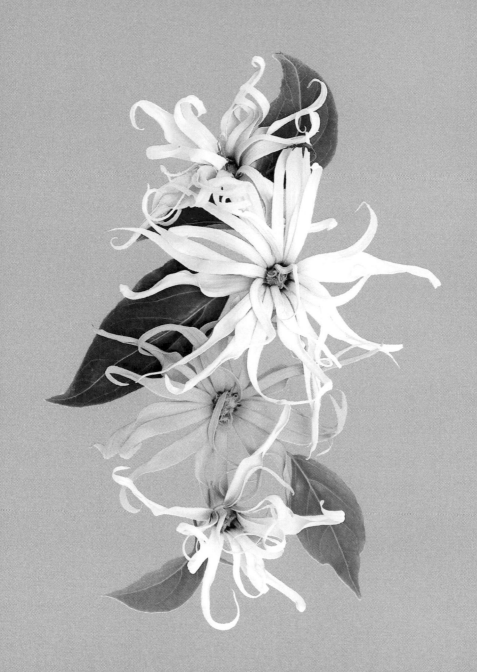

IMPROVING SLEEP AND DETOXIFYING THE BRAIN

Like other organs in the body, your brain needs to regularly clean house, eliminating cellular debris, metabolic waste, and toxic buildup. This detoxification effort can occur only while you are sleeping.

Sleep, Circadian Rhythms, and Melatonin

Restful sleep is critical for your health. This means falling asleep and staying asleep for at least eight hours a night and waking up feeling well rested and able to remember your dreams.

Your ability to fall asleep is related to sleep-wake cycles, known as circadian rhythms. Your pineal gland, located in the center of your brain, responds to these cycles and releases melatonin, a hormone that prepares you for sleep, as well as detoxifying your body and your brain. A lack of melatonin is almost always related to chronic disease, because without melatonin, your brain cannot detoxify, regenerate, and heal. Decreased production of melatonin is frequently found in patients with neurodegenerative diseases, such as Alzheimer's and Parkinson's.

Essential oils can be used to heal your pineal gland and trigger the natural release of melatonin, which helps your brain to detoxify and continue producing melatonin on its own.

What Is Melatonin?

Melatonin is your body's natural sleep hormone—it helps you shift from a waking state to a sleep state by regulating your circadian rhythms. The pineal gland begins to release melatonin when the sun goes down, peaking late in the evening, telling you that it is time to sleep. Melatonin levels fluctuate throughout the year, as the length of the night influences the duration of melatonin secretion.

Melatonin has been shown to help promote healthy sleep patterns, including reducing sleep latency (the amount of time needed to fall asleep), boosting sleep efficiency (the percentage of time in bed spent asleep), and increasing total sleep duration. Melatonin exerts both a hypnotic (sleep-inducing) and sedative (anxiety-relieving) effect to support your body's natural sleep-wake cycles.

Melatonin levels also shift with age. Most infants do not produce consistent levels of melatonin until the age of three months; this helps to explain why newborn sleep patterns can vary widely. During adolescence, melatonin patterns shift again. While most adults start to produce melatonin at about 10:00 p.m., teenagers release the sleep hormone later at night and thus tend to fall asleep later and feel groggy in the morning. Melatonin production decreases with age, correlating with an increase in chronic illness with age.

Primarily produced and released by the pineal gland, melatonin is also derived in the gut from the amino acid tryptophan and the neurotransmitter serotonin. Melatonin is fat-soluble, allowing it to easily travel throughout your brain and diffuse into cells to protect against damage.

Supplementation Versus Stimulation of Melatonin

Because melatonin is a hormone that your body produces naturally, supplementation should be used wisely. Not all forms of supplemental melatonin are able to cross the blood-brain barrier. Essential oils and liposomal melatonin remedies continually prove more effective in promoting sleep than melatonin consumed in pill form.

The effectiveness of essential oils in stimulating melatonin production could be due, in part, to the fact that melatonin is produced in plants and defends plant cells as an antioxidant. Melatonin serves a similar antioxidant function in humans and has been used to treat a number of health conditions and diseases, including insomnia, Alzheimer's disease, and depression.

MELATONIN SUPPORTS SLEEP

Research has proven melatonin to be an effective treatment for several of the following sleep-related issues.

Insomnia. Melatonin provides relief from the inability to fall asleep and stay asleep (insomnia) by reducing how long it takes you to fall asleep and improving total sleep time, sleep quality, and daytime alertness.

Jet lag. Melatonin can help prevent and reduce jet lag symptoms, promoting alertness, particularly when traveling east, since it resets your body's circadian rhythms, helping you adapt to local time.

Shift-work disorder. Melatonin might improve daytime sleep quality and duration in people whose jobs require them to work outside the traditional morning-to-evening schedule.

Sleep-wake cycle disturbances. Melatonin has been shown to support sleep disturbances in children.

Delayed sleep disorder. Melatonin can help reset sleep patterns, including disorders where sleep patterns are delayed, causing you to go to sleep later and wake up later. Melatonin can both advance the start of sleep and reduce the length of time needed to fall asleep.

OTHER HEALTH BENEFITS

Helping you get a good night's sleep so your brain can detoxify makes melatonin a hormone superstar. But that's not all this amazing chemical messenger does to keep your body healthy. As an antioxidant, melatonin is an effective "scavenger" that detoxifies the body, one cell at a time. This process takes place in many parts of the body, particularly in the eyes, bone marrow, brain, and digestive and reproductive organs. Melatonin protects brain tissue, repairing damage to your brain and guarding the nervous system against neurodegenerative diseases, such as Alzheimer's, Parkinson's, ALS or Lou Gehrig's disease, and even debilitating migraines.

Melatonin serves many of the following important functions in the body:

Increases antioxidant protection. Melatonin protects your cells and tissues by binding to and neutralizing substances that cause cellular damage. For example, free radicals are molecules that lack electrons, which makes them unstable. They steal electrons from other molecules and damage your cells in the process. Antioxidants act as a natural "off" switch for these free radicals by giving up some of their own electrons and breaking the damaging chain reaction. Melatonin serves as the strongest antioxidant in your body (with twice the antioxidant power of vitamin E), helping to regulate and repair cell damage.

Enhances immune function. Melatonin stimulates your immune system by supporting healthy cells and preventing unhealthy cells (like cancer) from forming in the first place. Melatonin has also been shown to slow the progression of advanced-stage cancers and decrease treatment side effects.

Supports detoxification. Melatonin can help your brain detoxify from chemicals, viruses, bacteria, mycotoxins (from mold), parasites and their toxic by-products, as well as heavy metals such as mercury, lead, aluminum, cadmium, and even fluoride, which can impair the function of the pineal gland. Melatonin, when released in healthy levels, will bind to heavy metals and reduce their toxicity.

Supports your gallbladder. High concentrations of melatonin are found in your bile. Melatonin has many gallbladder supportive properties, such as converting cholesterol to bile and increasing the mobility of gallstones from the gallbladder.

Activates brain regeneration. Research shows that melatonin activates proteins in the brain that regenerate nerve cells.

Impacts cardiovascular health. Research indicates that melatonin has a positive impact on cardiovascular health, including your heart and blood pressure.

Strengthens the blood-brain barrier. Melatonin has been found to support the barrier between the blood and the brain, keeping harmful substances out while allowing vital nutrients to reach the brain.

Offers neuroprotection. Healthy levels of melatonin help prevent and decrease cognitive decline. It is believed to protect brain cells from a protein called beta-amyloid, which is thought to contribute to Alzheimer's disease. Melatonin is so neuroprotective that administering it to stroke victims may limit brain tissue damage and prevent negative consequences like behavioral deficits or even death.

Reduces inflammation. Melatonin's antioxidant effect reduces tissue destruction and organ damage from inflammation. Melatonin has been shown to prevent and reduce the upregulation of pro-inflammatory cytokines, which can help to reduce brain swelling and brain cell death.

Supports mitochondrial function. Melatonin serves as effective protection against toxins that attack the mitochondria—the cells' power centers—and helps restore cells to their full function.

Alleviates migraines. Research published by the American Academy of Neurology in the journal *Neurology* suggests that the anti-inflammatory effect of melatonin reduces the frequency and severity of migraines. More than two-thirds of those in the study experienced at least a 50 percent reduction in the number, intensity, and duration of headaches per month.

Reduces symptoms of tinnitus. Melatonin may help reduce symptoms of tinnitus, a condition characterized by a constant ringing in the ears. Research by doctors published in the *Journal of Physiology* *and Pharmacology* found melatonin to be 150 times more effective at decreasing tinnitus symptoms than drugs designed to treat the condition.

Reduces depression. Because melatonin helps regulate your circadian rhythm, it can reduce symptoms of seasonal depression in fall and winter, when the days are shorter. Melatonin also reduced symptoms of treatment-resistant depression by 20 percent, according to a study on seasonal affective disorder (SAD) published in the journal *Psychiatry.*

Supports eye health and vision. Your eyes produce melatonin when exposed to light. Melatonin, in turn, helps protect your retinas and lowers the risk of eye-related diseases such as glaucoma. Low levels of melatonin in early development can contribute to vision problems.

Stabilizes blood pressure. Research has found that melatonin significantly decreased nighttime blood pressure, without modifying heart rate.

Balances blood sugar. Diabetes and diabetic neuropathies are linked with low levels of melatonin. Melatonin improves liver function (which helps balance blood sugar) and protects cells against insulin resistance and diabetes.

Supports gut health. Melatonin, in combination with the hormone prolactin, helps to balance gut flora, regenerate a healthy gut lining, and support healthy bowel function.

Protects the stomach by reducing ulcers and Gastroesophageal Reflux Disease (GERD). Melatonin may help heal stomach ulcers and alleviate heartburn. It strengthens your lower esophageal sphincter, blocking the secretion of stomach acids that contribute to ulcers and GERD, a condition caused by the backflow of stomach acid into the esophagus.

Regulates hormones. Melatonin controls body temperature and female reproductive hormones by inhibiting the release of certain hormones from the pituitary gland. Healthy melatonin levels optimize fertility and support ovarian health, egg quality, and production. Melatonin increases the levels of Human Growth Hormone (HGH), which supports weight loss and cellular regeneration.

Benefits those with autism. Children with autism have abnormal melatonin pathways and below-average physiological levels of melatonin. Enhancing melatonin production improves their ability to detoxify metals like aluminum, which can vastly improve health and mood.

Slows hair loss. Clinical studies on the topical application of melatonin showed a significant reduction in hair loss related to aging and medical conditions, like alopecia and dermatitis. Melatonin application also improved hair condition and texture and led to new hair growth in some cases.

How Melatonin Cleans the Brain

Your cell's waste disposal system relies on cell components called lysosomes, which are filled with enzymes that break down unwanted waste and materials. Lysosomes cannot perform their important clearing work without sulfate, a sulfur compound that helps clear cellular debris.

Your pineal gland produces melatonin in the evening, and melatonin delivers sulfate to various parts of the brain during sleep to clear cellular debris. Sulfate also helps to make the fat-loving molecules of melatonin more water-soluble, so they can move through your cerebrospinal fluid for delivery into the brain.

Dr. Stephanie Seneff, a senior research scientist at the MIT Computer Science and Artificial Intelligence Laboratory, has identified an insufficient supply of sulfate as the root cause of many neurological diseases. A lack of sulfate in the brain may impair your brain's ability to eliminate heavy metals and other toxins, resulting in an accumulation of cellular debris. Toxic metals and glyphosate (an herbicide) interfere with sulfate synthesis, and their effects accumulate over time.

Circadian Rhythms and the Sleep-Wake Cycle

Circadian rhythms are the cycles that tell your body when to sleep, wake, and eat. Every process in your body, from sleep to digestion and detoxification, follows a rhythmic or repetitive pattern based on twenty-four hour cycles. Your circadian rhythm regulates the signals that make you feel tired, sleep, wake up, and feel alert around the same time each day.

This internal clock regulates key organs and systems, including your heart, lungs, immune system, and metabolism, as well as patterns of brain-wave activity, hormone production, cell regeneration, and DNA repair.

Your body increases the responses to stimuli, like metabolism and self-defense functions, during the hours it expects to need them and down-regulates them during periods of rest. During the active phase of the day, bile acids and nutrient transporters are more active, as is energy metabolism. Conversely, detoxification becomes more active during the rest phase. This helps explain why some physical and mental activities seem easier at certain times of the day and may impact the best times to eat meals or take supplements.

CIRCADIAN RHYTHM DISRUPTIONS

The following symptoms may indicate an imbalance in your circadian rhythm:

- Inability to fall asleep
- Inability to stay asleep
- Difficulty waking up in the morning
- Not feeling refreshed after sleep
- Delayed recovery after physical activity
- Drop of energy between 4:00 and 7:00 p.m.
- Headache only during certain parts of the day

Shift work, travel through different time zones, staying up all night, and exposure to artificial light can disrupt your body's natural circadian rhythm, throwing off your sleeping, waking, and digestive systems and increasing the risk of health problems that include:

- Allergies
- Asthma
- Cardiovascular disease
- Hypertension
- Insomnia
- Digestive or metabolic disorders
- Anxiety and depression
- Stroke

Restoring healthy circadian rhythms and melatonin levels can take time, but it is worth the wait. Disruptions in your circadian rhythms reduce life expectancy, and age makes you more sensitive to these disruptions.

The Pineal Gland and Your Health

Your pineal gland is a pea-sized pinecone-shaped endocrine gland, located at eye level in the center of the brain. Acting as the "regulator of regulators," the pineal gland plays a role in every aspect of body functioning, including reproductive function, executive functioning, growth, body temperature, blood pressure, motor activity, sleep, mood, hormone regulation, immunity, and longevity.

The pineal gland influences the secretion of other chemical messengers, including neurotransmitters, endorphins, hormones, and dimethyltryptamine (DMT), a catalyst for higher states of consciousness and intuition linked to the "third eye" moniker for the pineal gland.

When your eyes' retinas detect darkness, they signal your pineal gland to release melatonin, telling your body to prepare for sleep. Dissected pineal glands revealed the presence of a photoreceptor, a structure activated by light.

Your pineal gland is the most vulnerable part of your brain—any toxin, stressor, or electromagnetic field that is affecting you will strongly affect your pineal gland, which then compromises melatonin production and with it your health. The pineal gland is so sensitive to chemicals that it is hypothesized that exposure to modern toxins has shrunk the pineal gland. Indian masters of the Vedic period were believed to have had a pineal gland the size of a lemon. Today, the pineal gland is the size of a small pea.

The symptoms of a compromised pineal gland include:

——— Mental health issues, particularly seasonal symptoms
——— Depression
——— Anxiety
——— Mood disorders, including paranoia, pessimism, and anger
——— Neurological disorders, including dementia, epilepsy, and Parkinson's disease
——— Hormonal issues, including changes in fertility, menstrual cycle, and ovulation
——— Impaired circadian rhythms, including sleeping too much or too little, feeling active and restless in the middle of the night, and feeling sleepy at unusual times
——— Not remembering dreams
——— Tendency to over-analyze
——— Headache, nausea, and vomiting
——— Difficulty with sense of direction or a feeling of spaciness
——— Difficulty losing weight

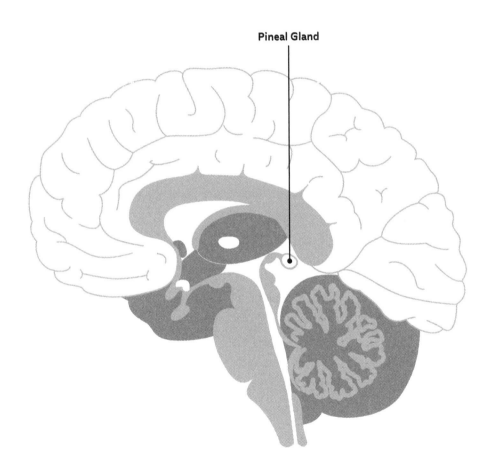

Pineal Gland

ENVIRONMENTAL TOXINS CAN HARM THE PINEAL GLAND

Unlike most of the brain, the blood-brain barrier doesn't protect your pineal gland. Instead, the pineal receives a tremendous amount of blood flow, second only to the kidneys, making it highly susceptible to the following environmental toxins that synergistically combine to damage your pineal gland:

Aluminum. Found in many foods, pharmaceuticals, personal-care products, and some vaccines, aluminum is toxic to your brain. It can damage your pineal gland and its ability to produce melatonin and contribute to degenerative diseases like Alzheimer's, Parkinson's, ALS, or Lou Gehrig's disease. Aluminum impairs your pineal gland's ability to detoxify and eliminate metals, creating a vicious cycle, where metals are more easily absorbed into the brain. When melatonin levels are optimal, melatonin binds to heavy metals, reducing their toxicity by helping you dispose of them.

Fluoride. Found in drinking water and toothpaste, fluoride is a toxic chemical by-product of manufacturing. It is a fat-soluble neurotoxin that accumulates in the pineal gland, creating a hard shell of phosphate crystals around the pineal called calcification. Pineal calcification jeopardizes melatonin production and accelerates neurodegenerative diseases and aging. Up to 60 percent of the population may experience pineal gland calcification.

Glyphosate. This active ingredient in the herbicide Roundup is associated with low melatonin levels. Glyphosate is believed to suppress melatonin synthesis by damaging gut microbes and depleting melatonin precursors like tryptophan and serotonin. Glyphosate increases aluminum toxicity by "caging" aluminum, allowing ingested aluminum to bypass the gut barrier and make it more accessible to the body. Glyphosate increases calcium uptake, allowing aluminum to gain entry to your cells by mimicking calcium. Aluminum then promotes calcium loss from the bones, contributing to pineal gland calcification.

Electromagnetic fields (EMFs). Exposure to EMFs can negatively impact the function of the pineal gland and suppress melatonin levels. It is suspected that the pineal gland senses EMFs as light, which may therefore decrease the melatonin production. Melatonin has been shown to be protective against EMFs, helping the pineal gland create more melatonin output, which protects against EMF damage.

HOW STRESS IMPACTS THE PINEAL GLAND

Melatonin, as a sleep hormone, has an antagonistic relationship to the stress hormone cortisol, which helps regulate alertness. This means that when cortisol is high, melatonin is low. That's fine during the day, but when cortisol levels are elevated at night, they turn off melatonin production and make it more difficult to fall asleep.

Chronic and prolonged stress triggers your adrenal glands to overproduce cortisol, throwing off your body's natural cortisol-melatonin rhythm. Cortisol levels should be highest in the morning when you wake up and gradually taper off throughout the day, so you feel tired at bedtime and can fall asleep. If you are active at night, especially in response to thought-driven stressors and anxiety, and slow in the morning, cortisol patterns are reversed.

A deficiency of sunlight or darkness, a poor diet, or ineffective absorption of food can compromise your pineal gland and impact your ability to produce melatonin. To help return your body to balance, it is important to detoxify and heal the pineal gland.

HEAL THE PINEAL GLAND AND RESTORE CIRCADIAN RHYTHM WITH ESSENTIAL OILS

Some people use a melatonin hormone supplement as a sleep aid. This may help in the short term, but it won't heal the pineal gland, which is supposed to make its own melatonin. Essential oils can help the pineal gland return to its innate intelligence and release more melatonin naturally. Activating the pineal gland with essential oils can help prevent and potentially reverse the damage from fluoride exposure and other environmental toxins.

Inhalation and topical or transdermal delivery of essential oils are more effective in activating the pineal gland to produce melatonin. The right oils can help trigger the natural release of melatonin and essentially guide the pineal gland back to its proper function. By healing the pineal gland, you will start sleeping more deeply; you will dream again and remember your dreams; and your memory will come back, your mental clarity and vitality will return, and you will make better decisions. When the proper level of melatonin begins circulating in your system, it will boost your ability to detoxify and address chronic illness and slow the aging process.

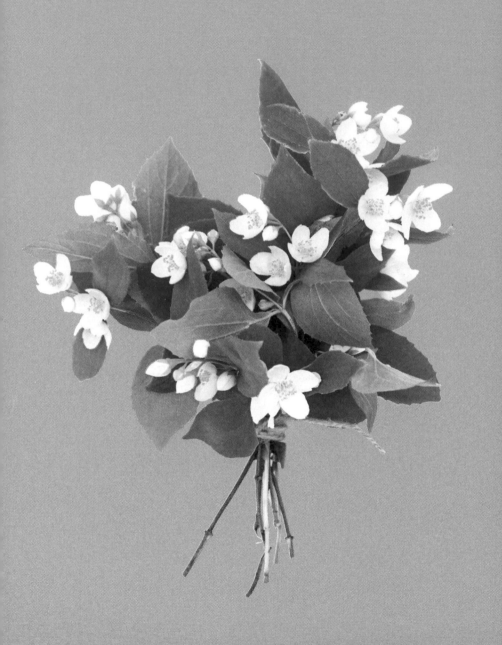

Brain Detoxification

Your brain detoxifies while you are sleeping through the glymphatic system, the waste clearance system for your brain that helps remove toxins and maintain brain health. Each night, during deep sleep, your brain literally shrinks, making room for cerebrospinal fluid to flow through and wash your brain, exiting down the lymphatic vessels in your neck, through the blood, to the liver, gallbladder, and intestines for elimination.

Removing Toxins through the Neck

While this is happening, the lymph system, in collaboration with the circulatory system, carries nutrients to the brain to repair the damage from toxins. This system keeps neurological degeneration and disease at bay and is one of the most underappreciated but vital mechanisms in your body.

It is also a system that is delicate and easily injured and upset. If any of those functions are impaired or congested, metabolic garbage builds up in the brain, contributing to degenerative diseases. For example, the buildup of beta-amyloid protein is believed to contribute to Alzheimer's disease, because the excess beta-amyloid clumps together and forms plaques that collect between the brain cells and disrupts cell communication and function.

Supporting brain detoxification is one of the most important things you can do for your health. This means both getting optimal sleep, so the brain can shrink and get washed, and ensuring that the exit route for the toxins—your neck—is not congested, so toxins can leave the brain. Elimination pathways in your body (blood, liver, gallbladder, and gut) also need to be open and flowing to avoid a backup of fluid that prevents toxins from leaving the body.

You might think of the body like a hydraulic system, where congested tissue downstream (like in the liver or the gut) prevents optimal flow upstream (from the brain flowing down). More specifically, congested lymphatic vessels in the neck or further down in the body can backlog the drainage of toxins from the brain.

Imagine thousands of fans trying to leave a parking lot after a sporting event or concert. If one car near the exit stops moving (due to a dead battery or another issue), it prevents all the cars behind it from moving as well. This is what happens in your body. If you are constipated and not able to eliminate toxins from your intestines, it backs up the toxic flow through the gallbladder, liver, and lymph system and into the brain.

OPENING DRAINAGE PATHWAYS WITH ESSENTIAL OILS

The compounds in essential oils help keep plants healthy by moving vital fluids and energy. They transport water from the roots to the leaves and perform similar functions in your body, helping to move energy, flush toxins like viruses and heavy metals, and prevent stagnation. Essential oils can help open drainage channels like those in your lymphatic and circulatory systems to improve the flow of energy and toxins through the blood, into the detoxification organs, and then out of the body.

A report in *Science* magazine reported that certain types of anesthetics, or substances that reduce sensitivity to pain, dramatically increase the space between your brain cells so fluid can flow more easily to help wash the brain.

Essential oils like clove, eucalyptus, lavender, fennel, black pepper, and peppermint have sedative and anesthetic properties. For example, the administration of clove oil, which is high in the constituent eugenol, dramatically decreased the time required for the induction of anesthesia. Similarly, both fenchone, a constituent of fennel essential oil, and linalool, a naturally occurring constituent in lavender oil, have acute local analgesic effects.

How the Brain Detoxifies

The brain has two main methods of detoxification: one is melatonin (see page 51), and the other is the glymphatic system, which physically clears waste and cellular garbage, including beta-amyloid—the protein associated with Alzheimer's disease—from the brain.

THE GLYMPHATIC SYSTEM

The glymphatic system is a waste clearance pathway in the brain that was discovered in 2012. The name glymphatic, or glial-dependent lymphatic system, is derived from the glial cells (brain immune cells) that work in combination with the lymphatic system to move cerebrospinal fluid across the brain tissue in a sweeping motion, washing brain cells and carrying debris down the neck and out of the body via lymph vessels that run parallel to your vagus nerve.

The glymphatic system not only serves as a pathway for clearing waste from the brain but it also helps distribute nutrients throughout the brain and circulates hormones like norepinephrine, which contributes to cognitive health.

While you sleep, your brain shrinks to allow increased space for cleaning fluid controlled by the lymphatic system to move through the pathways in and around the brain to speed up the removal of toxins and waste. Your brain needs to be in the deep sleep state in order to disengage and enable glymphatic function. During waking hours, your brain is actively working and cannot shut off to allow for a deep cleaning.

This system can become overloaded and slow down as we age, contributing to a buildup of metabolic garbage between the cells that contributes to inflammation and neurodegenerative diseases. Healthy glymphatic function can prevent or repair cognitive decline. This means both getting optimal sleep, so the brain can shrink and get washed, and ensuring that the exit route for the toxins—your neck—is not congested.

NECK CONGESTION IMPEDES TOXIN DRAINAGE

Your neck is the critical intersection where your brain connects with your body. Oxygen, nutrients, and signals are carried between the brain and the body through the nerves, lymph, blood vessels, and spinal cord that travel through your neck. (See page 67.)

Congestion in the neck impedes movement—the good things can't get in, and the bad things can't get out. Any inflammation in the vagus nerve, lymph nodes, blood vessels, or muscles of the neck blocks movement in the other systems and prevents the glymphatic fluid from draining from the brain. Fresh oxygenated blood can only enter your brain if blood and lymph are flowing properly.

Congested lymph or blood flow in the neck causes fluid and pressure buildup in the brain. Further, if toxins are mobilized and can't leave the brain, they recirculate and relocate in the brain to a position where they may cause more inflammation and damage, contributing to symptoms like headaches, fatigue, brain fog, vertigo, dizziness, tinnitus, blurred vision, and shifts in mood like anxiety and depression.

What Is the Glymphatic System?

In order to understand what can throw off your glymphatic system, it's important to understand how your brain cells and lymphatic system collaborate to form a brain-based garbage disposal system.

Glial cells are your brain's immune cells that protect, nourish, and insulate neurons and help clear waste. A particular type of glial cell, known as astroglia, has receptors, called aquaporin-4 channels, that help facilitate fluid movement to drive the removal of waste from your brain. The presence of aquaporins helps regulate the flux of water into and out of cells, facilitating a three- to ten-fold increase in water permeability compared to simple diffusion.

Lymph is a colorless fluid that circulates around the body and clears excess fluids and waste products from the gap between cells that is referred to as the interstitial space. The waste travels down the neck, parallel to the arteries, into a network of channels, known as the lymphatic system, where bacteria and pathogens are neutralized and eliminated.

These two systems—the glial cells and lymphatic system—collaborate to move fluid in the brain and support the circulation of nutrients and neurotransmitters that help to support brain function and memory.

Chronic disease specialist Dr. Dietrich Klinghardt began taking ultrasounds of his patients' necks and noticed a distinct correlation between chronic illness and inflammation in the vagus nerve, lymphatic tissue, and blood vessels. Consequently, he prioritized opening the drainage pathways in the neck channel with essential oils and other topical remedies like castor oil and CBD oil and noticed a dramatic reduction in inflammation in the drainage pathways, including the vagus nerve, which correlates with improved health.

As discussed earlier in regard to vagus nerve health (see page 35), it's important to help ensure optimal function in the neck to help your brain drain and detoxify better and to improve the delivery of oxygen, nutrients, and

NECK CONGESTION IMPEDES DRAINING OF TOXINS

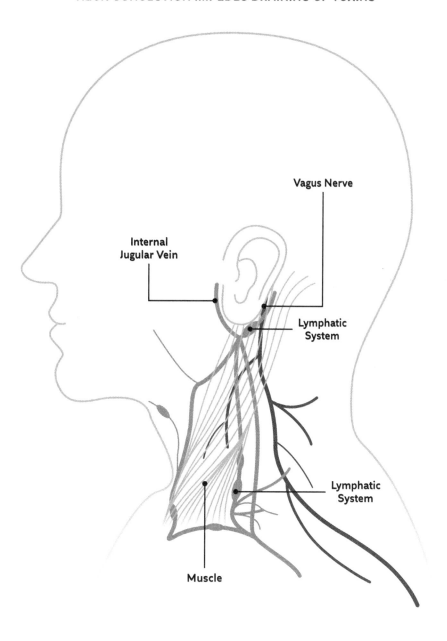

signals to your brain. Clearing congestion in the neck helps improve lymphatic flow, enhance circulation, and support healthy sinus and tonsil drainage.

Improving Lymphatic Flow

Your lymphatic system serves as your body's septic system, performing critical detoxification and immune functions. It draws excess fluid, toxins, and waste products from your cells and the spaces between the cells and carries them through a series of lymphatic ducts and nodes into your bloodstream, where they can be transported to the liver.

Your lymphatic system permeates every part of the body, transporting lymph—an infection-fighting fluid that circulates through a large network of tissues and organs via lymphatic vessels that then connect to lymph nodes (located in your tonsils, groin, spleen, and armpits), where toxins are filtered out. Your lymphatic system serves as a prefilter for the liver to prevent clogging and liver overload. Infections require your lymph nodes to work harder and filter out bacteria and viruses that can cause swelling. The lymphatic system also helps carry nutrients, oxygen, hormones, and other healing substances into every cell.

The lymphatic system can get congested and stagnant and toxins can build up. Unlike your cardiovascular system, your lymphatic system does not have a central pump—it only moves as the muscles squeeze it along. Any lack of movement stagnates the lymphatic system, with waste accumulating and excessive toxins building up. This stagnation can be due to an overload of acidity, animal protein, gluten, infection, toxins, or adhesions of the connective tissue, such as scars.

The more you can help the lymph fluid flow, the more quickly you can move toxins out of the body. Attempts to detoxify the body when the lymph system is congested often lead to discomfort and healing reactions—an adverse response to detoxification that presents as symptoms like headache, muscle pain, skin breakouts, and anxiety. Other symptoms of lymph congestion include fatigue, brain fog, swollen lymph nodes or tonsils, frequent colds, flu, sore throat, sinus congestion, constipation, and weight gain.

Essential oils can be used to help stimulate and amplify lymphatic flow and tissue fluid circulation. Peppermint and spearmint, in particular, are known for their cooling and anti-inflammatory properties that positively influence lymphatic flow, especially when used in combination with saunas, dry brushing the skin, and jumping on a trampoline.

Enhancing Circulation

The glymphatic system moves alongside the arteries and drains alongside the veins of the neck. Your circulatory system also controls blood flow into and out of the brain, harnessing the pulsing of blood in circulation to help keep things moving. The rhythmic expansion and contraction of blood flow through the veins and arteries help drive the movement of fluid draining from the brain. Slow or blocked blood flow through the veins or arteries can impede the ability of toxins to drain.

If veins and arteries are narrow, lax, scarred, or malformed, blood flow is restricted, which creates pressure and prevents toxins from draining from the brain. For example, conditions like high blood pressure cause blood vessels to lose their elasticity, becoming increasingly stiff. The regular pulsing of arterial walls drives the glymphatic system, so this stiffening impedes its function. In fact, researchers have demonstrated that high blood pressure–induced artery stiffening prevents the body from efficiently getting rid of large molecules in the brain, such as beta-amyloid. This finding might help explain the link between elevated blood pressure and cognitive decline and dementia.

Preventing Infections

Your veins can also be a target for infections. Inflammation in the veins of the neck caused by infections in the neck can restrict blood flow to and from the brain. As a result, blood backs up in the brain and spinal cord, which can trigger pressure and inflammation.

It has been proposed that viruses or parasites might hang out in the endothelium, or the lining, of the jugular vein and the venous system, causing congestion. Dr. Klinghardt notes, "If I were a bug, I would want to be waiting downstream from the most nutrient-rich blood in the body, and that's coming out of the brain." These infections can be addressed by taking the four steps below along with applying essential oils.

1   Keep the Vagus Nerve Healthy
    Your vagus nerve travels down both sides of the neck (see page 24), and infections in that vicinity can be taken into the nerve and contribute to inflammation that compromises the flow of fluids in the neck channel. Topically applying a combination of clove and lime essential oils on your vagus nerve can heal the infection and improve drainage.

2   Support Healthy Sinus and Tonsil Drainage
    Infections in the neck area, including your sinus cavity or tonsils, can inflame the neck and impede toxins from properly draining down the back of the throat when you swallow. If the sinus passages become blocked or fail to let the sinuses drain effectively, the resulting pressure can cause inflammation and congestion that is often correlated with neck pain.

Similarly, all waste that leaves the brain passes through the tonsils, which Dr. Klinghardt refers to as "the toilet of the brain." If your tonsils are congested or infected, they can act like a dam on the lymphatic system, preventing the glymphatic system of the brain from being able to properly drain. The tonsils are also in close proximity to and can infect your vagus nerve.

3 Reduce Toxicity in the Mouth
Oil pulling is a powerful tactic to literally "pull" toxins and bacteria from the mouth, attracting the fatty membranes of bacteria to the fat in the oil like a powerful magnet. Bacteria hiding in the crevices of your gums and within and between your teeth are sucked out of their hiding places and held firmly in the solution.

Oil pulling cleans your mouth like soap cleans dirty dishes. Swishing or holding 1 to 2 teaspoons of edible oil (like coconut oil or sesame oil) in your mouth and around your teeth and gums—similarly to how you might swish mouthwash—for 10 to 20 minutes will draw out these impurities and wash them from the mouth. The longer you push and pull the oil through your mouth, the more pathogens are pulled free, so be careful not to swallow any. Spit out the oil after 10 to 20 minutes.

You can optimize the benefits even more by adding essential oils like clove, cinnamon, or peppermint to your oil-pulling routine. For example, clove oil contains the active ingredient eugenol, which helps naturally numb and reduce pain and inflammation. A study published in the *Journal of Dentistry* found that eugenol is more effective at reducing pain, inflammation, and infection than an analgesic toothpaste.

Katie Wells at Wellness Mama, an online resource for healthy living topics, recommends creating essential oil-pulling chews by combining ½ cup of melted coconut oil with 30 drops of essential oils, then allowing them to harden in the freezer in silicone candy molds for daily consumption. You can pop a hardened oil candy in your mouth for 15 minutes before spitting out the oil without swallowing.

4 Align the Spine
To optimize the highway in and out of the brain, it's important to make sure that the cervical spine is aligned. Injuries including whiplash, concussions, or traumatic brain injury can negatively affect lymph drainage along with other health concerns, as your spinal cord is the main pathway connecting the brain and peripheral nervous system.

Similarly, structural issues like jaw alignment or misalignment in conditions like temporomandibular joint (TMJ) syndrome, or a pain in the jaw joint, can compromise lymphatic drainage. The pumping action of your jaw helps physically move glymphatic fluid every time you swallow. Grinding teeth or clenching your jaw at night is one way that your body attempts to overcompensate and help support drainage during sleep.

Tight muscles in the neck can both constrict the veins in the neck, causing impaired blood flow to the brain, and put pressure on nerves and impede the flow of signals.

Essential oil blends, like the Structural Alignment Blend (page 204), can be topically applied after chiropractic sessions to help hold and maintain the correction. This blend has been referred to as the "chiropractor in a bottle."

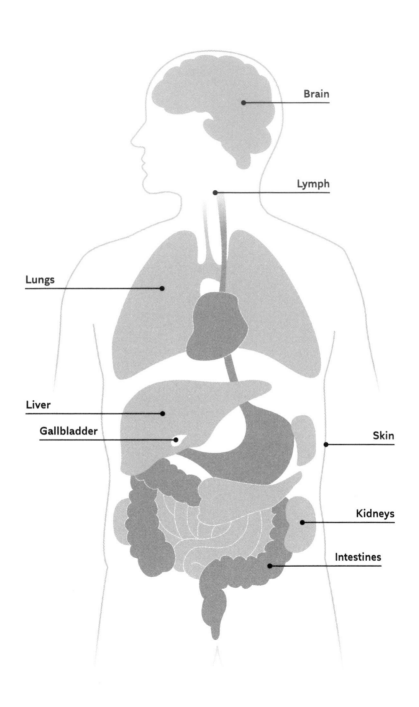

Brain

Lymph

Lungs

Liver

Gallbladder

Skin

Kidneys

Intestines

Detoxifying the Brain and Draining the Body

Fluids drain from your brain down through your body much like a stream flowing into a larger river and eventually into the ocean. As long as the waterway is open and not blocked by logs or sediment, everything flows smoothly. When there is a blockage in this flow, the water backs up and can flood the surrounding area and cause damage.

Once toxins draining from the brain clear the neck channel, they must continue to flow downstream in your blood, through your liver, to your gallbladder, and into your bile, which then transports toxins through the gut for elimination in your stool. As long as toxins flow in the right direction and do not encounter congested tissue or stagnation in any organ, they can be eliminated.

Congestion in your detoxification pathways, such as liver congestion or stagnant bile flow, impede the elimination of toxins. This pushes toxins back into your bloodstream where they are forced out through other detoxification pathways—your skin and your kidneys—leading to blemishes, scabs, and rashes, frequent urination, and lower back pain.

What Are Toxins?

Toxins can include any substance that creates an irritating or harmful effect in the body, including undigested food (think fats or proteins), excess hormones (like estrogen), and yeast overgrowth or other digestive concerns. Toxins can limit the ability of cells to function, so the body safely stores them in fat to avoid damage.

Some symptoms of toxicity in the body are fatigue, constipation, gas, bad breath, frequent infections, hormone imbalances, mood swings, depression, skin problems, poor circulation, and mucus buildup.

Essential oils possess specific properties that help support the detoxification process. The right blends of essential oils can:

——— Support organ function and vitality.
——— Improve the function of major elimination pathways by supporting the body's ability to clean tissues and eliminate waste.
——— Reduce inflammation.
——— Stimulate your white blood cells to help clean up toxins in the body.

OPENING DETOXIFICATION PATHWAYS WITH ESSENTIAL OILS

The detoxification pathways move the toxins out of the body. All of these pathways—including digestive, urinary, integumentary (skin), circulatory, respiratory, and lymphatic systems—must be open and flowing optimally, before you begin to mobilize toxins or kill pathogens. If the detoxification pathways are blocked or stagnant, mobilized toxins will likely be reabsorbed and you might feel even worse—as if you had the flu. This is often characterized as a "detox reaction" or "healing crisis," but what it really means is that the toxins are not leaving the body. If this happens, you may need to pause the detoxification effort and open the detoxification pathways.

Essential oils can play an especially powerful role in helping to open, enhance, and support the optimal function of these detoxification pathways. These oils are extremely gentle and can be topically applied, thus avoiding any additional burden on a potentially compromised digestive system. Essential oils help keep their plants healthy by moving vital fluids and energy through the plant. They perform similar functions in your body, helping to move fluids and prevent stagnation.

Topically applying essential oils to specific points on your skin can activate energy flow directly and quickly. The minute size of essential oil molecules allows them to be easily assimilated into the organs to help promote the directional flow of bile and toxins.

Aiding the Work of the Liver

Your liver is the most important player in your body's detoxification effort, filtering toxins from the blood and neutralizing the toxins in preparation for elimination. Essential oils that enhance liver function possess what are called hepatic properties. Liver tissue consists of a mass of hepatic cells, tunneled through with bile ducts and blood vessels that perform several metabolic functions. Supporting the vitality of your liver can dramatically enhance your ability to detoxify and heal. Essential oils that stimulate and tone your liver include carrot seed, German and Roman chamomile, cypress, grapefruit, ginger, helichrysum, juniper, lemon, peppermint, rosemary, spearmint, and turmeric (for more information, see page 179).

Expectorant for Your Lungs

Essential oils that help expel mucus out of your body and support your respiratory detoxification are known to possess expectorant properties. Essential oils that support respiratory detox include basil, cedarwood, clary sage, cypress, eucalyptus, frankincense, hyssop, marjoram, myrrh, myrtle, pine, Roman chamomile, rosemary, and sandalwood.

Laxative for Your Intestines

The gut is an important detoxification pathway to eliminate toxins from your body in your stool. Essential oils with laxative properties encourage bowel movements and promote detoxification of the intestines. Essential oils that stimulate the digestive process, bowel movement, and detoxification of the intestines include a combination of clove and lime, along with fennel, ginger, peppermint, rosemary, and spearmint.

Diaphoretic for Your Skin

Certain essential oils that support sweating and detoxification through your skin are called diaphoretic agents. Essential oils known to promote sweating include angelica, cinnamon, cardamom, clove, eucalyptus, German chamomile, ginger, helichrysum, peppermint, rosemary, spearmint, thyme, and yarrow.

Diuretic for Your Kidneys

Essential oils known to promote urination and elimination through the kidneys include black pepper, fennel, geranium, grapefruit, juniper, lemon, mandarin, and orange.

Emmenagogue for Your Uterus

An emmenagogue stimulates menstruation. Essential oils that promote healthy menstruation and carry toxins out of the body with blood flow include angelica, basil, cinnamon, clary sage, German and Roman chamomile, fennel, ginger, jasmine, juniper, lavender, marjoram, myrrh, peppermint, rose, and rosemary.

Promoting Biliary/Gallbladder Function

Essential oils, like blue tansy and black cumin, can help promote healthy bile flow and alleviate gallbladder congestion.

Lymphatic Enhancement

Essential oils that promote tissue-cleansing action of your lymphatic system include angelica, cypress, fennel, frankincense, geranium, grapefruit, juniper, lemon, palmarosa, peppermint, spearmint, vitex berry, and ylang-ylang. The cooling properties of mint, in particular, help enhance lymphatic flow. Castor oil also helps lymph flow and can be applied over your liver, on the sides of your neck, or on the bottoms of your feet in combination with essential oils.

Blood Purification

Essential oils can help purify and detoxify your blood, stimulating your white blood cells to clean up metabolic waste and toxins in your body. The process of cleaning out damaged cells, known as autophagy, helps you regenerate new healthy cells. Autophagy supports the lymphatic system to eliminate toxins, reduces inflammation induced by environmental irritants, toxins, and pathogens, and plays a role in cell communication, reprogramming your cells to return to health. Research has found that bergamot essential oil helps activate autophagy in your liver and your brain. Additional essential oils with blood purifying properties include cypress, fennel, grapefruit, juniper, lemon, and rosemary.

Autonomic Nervous System Activation

Stimulating the parasympathetic response also helps support the flow of bile to eliminate toxins. When the flow of bile is stagnant or slowed, your gut shifts toward a state of dysbiosis, where unfriendly flora dominate, and constipation is common. The toxins from pathogenic bacteria then block detoxification pathways in the liver as well. Activating the parasympathetic state helps calm inflammation that can impede detoxification and boosts healthy gut bacteria that help break down and eliminate toxins.

Inflammation Reduction

Essential oils can help calm and soothe inflammation in your body and your brain, which helps relieve tissue congestion and enhances the movement of toxins out of your body. Ginger essential oil, in particular, has been shown to have inflammatory-modulating properties. Other essential oils that help reduce inflammation include a blend of clove and lime along with a combination of dill, frankincense, ginger, grapefruit, tarragon, and ylang-ylang.

Unique properties of specific essential oils resonate with different organ systems, open detoxification pathways, and stimulate communication between your brain, liver, gallbladder, and gut for proper elimination.

The Liver

Your liver helps manage your energy by storing and releasing blood sugar, digesting food, and assimilating nutrients. It produces bile, which breaks down fats so they can be absorbed and carries wastes out in the stool. Your liver also synthesizes amino acids and contributes to bone and muscle growth.

An overload of toxins and stress can overwhelm your liver, impacting its ability to keep up with the toxic load. When the liver becomes sluggish and unable to process and eliminate toxins, they build up in your body, contributing to systemic toxicity, chronic inflammation, and the depletion of your nutrient reserves.

A liver detox typically involves modifying your diet to avoid foods that are harder for the liver to process (like sugar, caffeine, dairy, grains, and processed food). This detox gives your digestive system and your liver a break and allows it time to clear out the overload and rest. When you reduce the incoming toxic load, it allows the liver to catch up on the backlog of toxins. Essential oils can be powerful tools to open your detoxification pathways and detox the liver as well as strengthen, stimulate, and regenerate it.

SIGNS THAT YOUR LIVER IS OVERTAXED

Your liver lacks pain receptors, making it difficult to know when it's struggling and needs support. Since the liver is involved in so many functions of the body, symptoms of distress often manifest elsewhere, presenting as:

Excessive fatigue. Fatigue is common when the liver is under stress. The liver is responsible for managing blood sugar, which supports energy levels and combats fatigue. A stressed liver may become less efficient at regulating blood sugar, leading to fatigue and sugar cravings.

Estrogen imbalances or PMS. The liver helps balance hormone levels, detoxifying and eliminating excess estrogen. If liver function is impaired, excess estrogen may be reabsorbed, resulting in symptoms like premenstrual syndrome, breast tenderness, excessive bleeding, moodiness, and weight gain.

Bloating and gas. Poor liver function can compromise bile flow to your gut; this throws off the balance of good bacteria in your gut. The dominance of unfriendly gut flora contributes to constipation and keeps toxins from being eliminated, further contributing to gas and bloating.

Inability to process heavy metals. When the liver's detoxification pathways are impaired, heavy metals can accumulate in the body.

Chemical sensitivities and allergies. Your liver breaks down excess histamine. If your liver is sluggish, histamine can build up in your body, contributing to symptoms like a heightened sensitivity to smells, chemicals, and foods. Research shows that individuals with impaired bile flow have significantly higher levels of histamine in their blood.

Itchy skin. When your liver is impaired, it compromises optimal bile flow. The body then resorts to the skin for eliminating toxins, contributing to itchiness.

Bruising and bleeding. You may bruise more easily because the liver can no longer produce enough proteins to clot the blood after an injury. The liver actually produces several clotting factors, all of which begin to disappear when the liver is damaged.

Swelling. When the liver isn't able to do its job, your body may retain water in the abdomen and legs, causing swelling.

Poor sleep. Your liver filters and detoxifies harmful substances from the blood while you sleep, with heightened activity between 1:00 and 3:00 a.m. (often peaking at 3:00 a.m.). Waking up at this time often indicates liver overload.

Reactions to foods or drugs. In his book *The Toxin Solution*, Dr. Joseph Pizzorno suggests that any bad reaction to a food, drug, or toxin could indicate a need for increased liver support. These include adverse reactions to sulfite food additives (from salad bars, wine, or dried fruit), caffeine intolerance, a strong urine odor after eating asparagus, and feeling sick after eating garlic.

LIVER EMOTIONS

Your liver stores and releases "emotional toxins" that might present as:

- Feeling irritable or impatient
- Inappropriate anger, including angry outbursts
- Over-reactivity, flying off the handle, or having a difficult time letting things go
- Feelings of not feeling heard, not feeling loved, not being recognized, or an inability to be honest with yourself and others
- Experience of resentment, frustration, or bitterness
- Being judgmental, overly critical, finding fault, or complaining
- Feeling the need to control situations; being domineering or bossy

The Gallbladder

Your gallbladder is responsible for storing, releasing, and concentrating bile, a fluid produced in the liver that helps your body break down fat and carry toxins and old hormones out of the body. Ideally, your gallbladder releases this bile into your small intestine, where it breaks down the fat for your body to absorb, before being eliminated in the stool. When you eliminate the bile, you eliminate toxins with it. Unfortunately, chronic stress, toxicity, hormones, or diets too low or too high in fat can make your bile thick, viscous, and stagnant, impeding its ability to flow into the small intestine and out of the body.

If toxins do not exit your body, they can be reabsorbed, further adding to your body's toxic burden and contributing to hormonal imbalances and gallbladder challenges. Common symptoms of stagnant bile flow include motion sickness, mild headache above the eyes, pain between the shoulder blades, and signs of poor fat digestion like chronically dry skin and hair, floating stools, diarrhea, and/or greenish stools.

Black cumin seed essential oil is especially beneficial for the gallbladder and for restoring healthy bile flow, since the chemical constituent stearic acid in cumin seed is an ideal emulsifying agent that binds water and oil.

The Lymphatic System

Your lymphatic system serves as a complementary system to your circulatory system, transporting cellular and intercellular waste to the blood, where it can be processed and eliminated (for more information, see page 68). Essential oils such as spearmint and peppermint are some of the best tools to help stimulate and amplify lymphatic flow and tissue fluid circulation (see page 176).

The Intestines

Your intestines play an important role in detoxification and immune health, providing a physical barrier to stop pathogens from entering your body and maintaining a balance of good bacteria that assist in the maintenance of a balanced gut environment.

Normal detoxification during digestion depends on the integrity of the gastrointestinal membrane and the balance of the precise bacterial and chemical environment. An imbalance in the intestinal flora and injury to intestinal walls can allow undigested food and other contaminants to leak into the bloodstream. Similarly, regular and healthy bowel movements help toxins leave the body. Poor waste elimination is often correlated with toxins being reabsorbed into the body known as re-toxification. (For more information on the maintenance of your intestinal barrier, see page 188.)

The Skin

The skin is your largest organ and a major elimination pathway. Your body eliminates up to a pound of waste products every day through your skin. Your sweat glands act as a key channel, helping to support any toxic overflow from your liver or kidneys.

Skin reactions like acne, rosacea, psoriasis, rashes, or dry and itchy skin are often an indication that your liver and kidneys are processing more toxins than your body can handle. When your liver is unable to process toxins, your pores start to pitch in to sweat things out.

Sweat therapy can trace its roots to Native American sweat lodges, Scandinavian saunas, and Roman and Turkish baths. Recent research corroborates the benefits—toxins like heavy metals have been found in sweat after heavy exercise. Fat-soluble toxins, such as endocrine disruptors like bisphenol A (BPA), can escape in the sweat as well. Supporting the detoxification pathway through the skin can lessen the burden on other detoxification organs like the liver and the kidneys. This is especially helpful for the kidneys, since they are delicate organs and can be easily damaged by overuse.

Detox Bath

My favorite tool for eliminating toxins via sweat therapy is a detox bath (see full recipe on page 180) with Epsom salt, baking soda, and a few drops of either lavender or clove essential oil. The clove helps to pull toxins out of the skin to lessen the burden on the liver, gallbladder, and kidneys. But remember, oil and water don't mix! Blend the oils into the salt first to ensure their distribution in the water. Make the water as hot as you can tolerate and try to soak for at least 20 minutes, ideally three or four times weekly.

The Kidneys

Your kidneys are two bean-shaped organs that play a vital role in detoxification, filtering the blood and helping remove waste from the body through urination. When your liver is overworked, your kidneys take up the slack.

The kidneys also regulate the balance of fluids in the body, blood pressure (by maintaining the salt and water balance), and the body's acid-alkaline balance or pH (by selectively filtering out or retaining various minerals and electrolytes). The kidneys control the volume, composition, and pressure of fluids in all the cells. Blood flows through the kidneys at its highest pressure, filtering out toxins and directing nourishing materials to where they are needed.

When your kidneys overwork, you can experience symptoms like lower back pain, the need to urinate more frequently, puffiness around your eyes, and swollen feet and ankles.

If your skin and kidneys are not able to pick up the slack for your liver, your body will store toxins in fat cells to protect itself from those toxins flowing back to critical organs like your brain. When this occurs, you may experience weight gain, fatigue, and brain fog. The body will do anything it can, including adding extra weight to your frame, to move toxins out of your bloodstream to protect vital organs.

FUELING YOUR BRAIN WITH ENERGY TO HEAL

Just like a car, your brain needs fuel to run properly.
Brain fuel is oxygen, glucose (or blood sugar), and stimulation.
The brain needs a healthy supply of oxygen and nutrient-rich
blood to function properly, and it contains the densest network
of blood vessels carrying oxygen in your body. Although your
brain accounts for less than 2 percent of your total body weight,
it consumes approximately 20 percent of your body's oxygen
intake. This high oxygen demand makes your brain susceptible
to damage, when brain oxygen levels are compromised.

Circulation

Are your feet so cold that you need to wear socks to bed? Do you experience occasional memory lapses or brain fog? Perhaps you've noticed varicose veins or tingling in your hands or feet. All of these can be signs of poor circulation or a lack of blood flow and nutrients to extremities, like your hands, feet, and brain.

Your circulatory system consists of your heart, blood, arteries, and veins. Healthy circulation is critical for the delivery of oxygen and nutrient-rich blood to your brain, while simultaneously carrying toxins and waste to the kidneys and liver to be eliminated. An easy way to assess healthy circulation is to compare the temperature of your body to the temperature of your distal extremities like your fingers and toes as well as the tip of your nose. Essential oils can help support circulation by maintaining healthy heart rate variability, blood flow, and blood pressure.

Improving Blood Flow to Your Brain

Your circulatory system controls blood flow into and out of the brain. Brain cells will die without a healthy supply of oxygen-rich blood, but blood needs to flow against gravity to reach your brain.

Other challenges that can impact healthy blood flow to the brain include blood pressure or blood sugar that is too high or too low, smoking, alcoholism, chronic inflammation, hypothyroidism, diabetes, anemia, chronic stress, and advanced age.

Since your brain does not have pain receptors, symptoms of poor blood and oxygen flow often present as mental fatigue, including difficulty concentrating, poor memory, and depression. Symptoms of poor blood flow in the body including cold hands, feet, and face; poor nail health; thinning hair;

BLOOD FLOW TO YOUR BRAIN

The circulatory system controls blood flow into and out of the brain. Brain cells require a healthy supply of oxygen-rich blood.

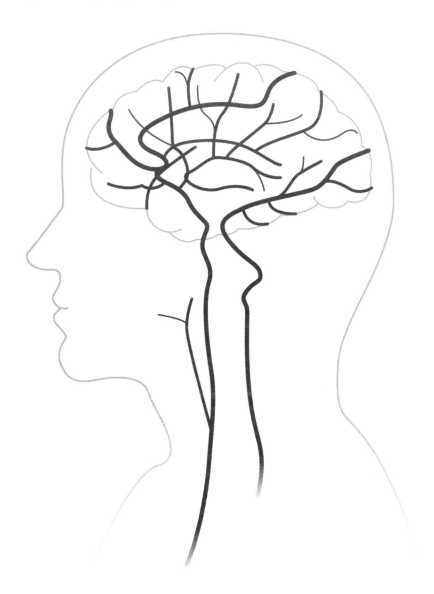

and erectile dysfunction—all indications that blood flow to the brain is likely compromised. Other symptoms include headaches, vertigo, dizziness, and insomnia. Poor brain blood flow and circulation can be linked to a number of medical conditions, including:

- Cognitive dysfunction and brain fog
- Chronic fatigue syndrome
- Dementia
- Parkinson's disease
- Alzheimer's disease
- Depression
- Post–traumatic stress disorder (PTSD)
- Anxiety
- Obsessive-compulsive disorder (OCD)
- Panic disorder
- Traumatic brain injury
- Lyme disease

THE HEALING POWER OF OXYGEN

Oxygen helps expedite your body's healing process. Increasing your brain's available oxygen through increased blood flow can improve your mood, energy, and mental clarity, while reducing your risk of dementia. It helps increase energy production, reduce brain inflammation, and improve reaction time for cognitive function. It's not surprising that pharmaceutical drugs designed to improve brain function often enhance blood flow to the brain and improve the brain's ability to utilize oxygen. Any kind of injury to your brain, including concussions and traumatic brain injury, require good circulation to enhance healing.

INCREASE BRAIN OXYGEN WITH ESSENTIAL OILS

Essential oils have been shown to increase circulation and blood flow to the brain. For example, essential oils can help relax and improve the health of your blood vessels (see pages 177–178). This helps more blood circulate through them, improving your circulation and increasing brain oxygen levels in the process.

Essential oils can be used to help your veins contract, stimulating blood flow. They may help reduce some of the buildup of triglycerides that can form and restrict blood flow. Essential oils can also be used to improve lymphatic system functionality that can help flush out toxins and reduce inflammation of the blood vessels, improving blood flow throughout the body.

What's more, essential oils that are high in sesquiterpenes—including black pepper, cedarwood, frankincense, ginger, myrrh, patchouli, sandalwood, spikenard, and vetiver—may help oxygenate your brain. Sesquiterpines are carbon chains that do not contain oxygen molecules but seem to pull oxygen in. This may be one reason why essential oils high in sesquiterpines increase oxygen levels in the brain when inhaled or topically applied to the skin around the head.

The Benefits of Black Pepper

Black pepper and its active compound piperine have been found to enhance circulation, increasing blood flow to your digestive system, which helps boost nutrient absorption. Piperine helps stimulate digestive enzymes, enhances digestive capacity, increases absorption in the intestines, and also significantly reduces gastrointestinal food transit times.

This means that your cells are better able to utilize nutrients and healing remedies when piperine is added, so much so that it is often added to supplement formulations to enhance the effectiveness of the supplement. Dr. Datis Kharrazian, a Harvard-trained clinical researcher, found that adding black pepper to his supplement formulations increased the absorption 200 to 400 percent.

Piperine has been shown to improve brain function in animal studies, perhaps due to its brain oxygenation properties. Piperine was found to improve memory in rats, allowing them to repeatedly run a maze more efficiently than rats who were not given the compound. In another rodent study, piperine extract seemed to decrease the formation of amyloid plaques, which are dense clumps of damaging protein fragments in the brain that have been linked to Alzheimer's disease. Black pepper also contains copious amounts of limonene, a naturally occurring terpene that can help dissolve cholesterol, which can clog veins and congest blood flow.

Blood Sugar

Carbohydrates in the food you eat are digested and absorbed as glucose, which is then transported through your bloodstream, supplying energy to every cell in your body. The body is continuously monitoring the levels of glucose in your blood so it doesn't spike too high or dip too low. The goal is to maintain a condition of internal stability for optimal function.

Blood sugar provides your brain with the energy it needs to function. Your brain is rich in nerve cells, or neurons, which have an incredibly high energy requirement. Your brain demands more energy from sugar than other organs—up to a third of the energy your body produces.

Your brain needs a continuous and permanent supply of glucose from your blood to support mental energy and brain signaling and to prevent neuro-degeneration. Thinking, memory, and learning are closely linked to glucose levels and how efficiently your brain uses that glucose. For example, neurons are excited or inhibited by the rise and fall of glucose levels in your brain. These neurons help control your metabolism and energy expenditure. Your brain needs more glucose to support a brain injury or compromised function. If that increased demand for energy cannot be met, brain function declines.

Improving Blood Sugar Balance Enhances Brain Function

Supplying your brain with the energy it needs to operate can be a delicate balancing act. When blood sugar is low, not enough glucose gets to the brain, and your brain will degenerate and not function well. If there isn't enough glucose in the brain, your brain's neurotransmitters, or chemical messengers, cannot communicate effectively. Similarly, when neurons lose the ability to use glucose efficiently as a fuel, brain cells begin to atrophy. Low blood sugar reduces power to the brain—it's like turning off your brain's battery.

If your energy levels change with your meals, it may indicate a blood sugar imbalance. If energy and focus are enhanced after eating, you are likely dealing with low blood sugar. If eating makes you feel lethargic or fatigued, you likely have high blood sugar. Unstable blood sugar can trigger brain symptoms like exhaustion, insomnia, anxiety, depression, and brain fog.

Similarly, constant fluctuation in blood sugar levels can throw your body into a state of chronic stress, adding fuel to your body's inflammatory fire. Excess blood sugar can result in chronically high levels of the stress hormone cortisol, which can trigger an increased production of inflammatory proteins associated with a heightened immune response. High cortisol levels also damage and atrophy an area of the brain known as the hippocampus, which plays an important role in memory and brain function. Stabilizing brain blood sugar helps to alleviate many autoimmune, inflammatory, and brain-based disorders.

LOW BLOOD SUGAR

When your blood sugar is low, your brain doesn't get enough fuel, contributing to poor brain function and endurance, impacting attention and cognitive function. This might make you feel spacey, lightheaded, shaky, or irritable.

If you go too long without eating, your brain can't get enough fuel to function properly. Skipping meals, eating less than normal, or exercising more than usual can lead to low blood sugar. If you get "hangry" (that is, hungry plus angry) between meals or feel physically and mentally better after you eat, you are likely dealing with low blood sugar.

HIGH BLOOD SUGAR

High blood sugar can trigger an inflammatory response, making you feel lethargic or drowsy, contributing to feelings of depression, anxiety, or irritability. Dr. Robert Atkins, an American physician and cardiologist best known for his bestselling *Atkins Diet,* talks about how sugar ages your body—damaging skin, nerves, eyes, joints, and arteries—at an accelerated pace. Atkins notes that sugar is "sticky." When you have extra sugar floating around in your bloodstream, those sticky glucose molecules attach themselves to proteins, forming advanced glycation end products (AGEs), which are related to the stiffening and loss of elasticity found in aging tissues.

When glucose attaches to a protein in places where it doesn't belong, it sets in motion a chain of chemical reactions, where proteins bind together and create a new structure. By altering the structure of proteins, their function is also altered. You might visualize what happens when you toast a piece of bread: it hardens because the sugars have bound under the gluten, another example of glycation. This hardening and altering of function occur in your collagen, the flexible connective tissue that holds your skeleton together. As collagen's flexibility is destroyed, your skin sags and your organs stiffen.

High levels of sugar in the blood mean sugar stays in the blood for too long, where it can bind to and damage your blood vessels and constrict blood flow to your brain. Specifically, high blood sugar reduces the production of nitrous oxide, a substance that helps to dilate or expand blood vessels, and increases the production of hormones that constrict blood vessels.

This is especially noticeable in your tiniest arteries like those in your eyes, contributing to eye damage, and in your kidneys, contributing to impaired kidney function. Your kidneys are designed to take these proteins that have been bound to sugar out of your system. If the kidneys must flush out extra glucose, you may experience symptoms like frequent urination and excessive thirst. Your body must release sugar through the urine, and it demands extra liquid to rehydrate.

AGEs also bind to cell membranes, where chemical signals are sent and received, impeding the ability of cell communication. They also bind to "bad" cholesterol (LDL), damaging the surfaces of your arteries. High levels of blood sugar actually *age* you, since AGEs are predictive of your longevity.

Causes of High Blood Sugar

Foods with a high sugar content or carbohydrates spike blood sugar. Increasing the intake of healthy fats and supporting the body's ability to digest and assimilate fats can help curb hunger cravings and sustain blood sugar levels.

Stress contributes to high blood sugar. Your body needs more glucose to fuel the demands of mental, emotional, or physical stress. Long-term stress requires the constant release of glucose into the bloodstream. This exhausts your adrenals (from releasing cortisol to stimulate the release of glucose reserves), your liver (from converting protein to glucose), and your pancreas (from releasing the hormone insulin to carry sugar out of your blood and into your cells) and exacerbates high blood sugar levels.

Environmental toxins block the receptor sites on the cells, preventing cells from properly assimilating glucose. In his book *The Toxin Solution*, Dr. Joseph Pizzorno specifically notes that toxins damage cell membranes, preventing them from getting important messages, such as insulin not signaling cells to absorb more sugar.

Insulin grabs glucose out of the bloodstream and carries it into your cells. You might think of insulin as the key that unlocks the cell receptor to allow glucose into your cells. When glucose levels in your bloodstream are too high, your pancreas secretes insulin to carry the sugar out of your bloodstream and into your cells, where excess blood sugar is converted into fat for storage. Over time, your cells can become overwhelmed by insulin and fail to properly respond, developing a resistance to the constant onslaught of insulin, known as insulin resistance.

The Effects of Insulin Resistance

When you develop insulin resistance, it is almost as if you are surrounded by water but unable to drink. Your blood becomes full of sugar, but it cannot be carried into your cells. Many bacteria, viruses, and fungi like to feed off of the high level of sugars in your blood. This is one reason diabetics, who have notoriously high blood sugar levels, are predisposed to so many infections—the excess sugar in the bloodstream attracts pathogens.

Despite the surplus of sugar in your bloodstream, your cells begin to starve. Your body tries to make more and more insulin in an attempt to overcome the cells' resistance to absorbing and using the insulin, which deprives them of energy. At the same time, too much sugar and insulin circulate throughout your bloodstream, contributing to inflammation and throwing off hormones and neurotransmitters that negatively impact your brain. High insulin levels also lower two other important hormones—glucagon and growth hormone—that are responsible for burning fat and sugar and promoting muscle development.

A common symptom of insulin resistance is becoming extremely sleepy after eating. This is due to the effects of the excess sugar and insulin surge on the brain's neurotransmitters, as well as the high-energy demand of converting sugar into fat. Insulin's key function in your brain is helping it utilize glucose, so when the brain becomes resistant to insulin, it does not properly assimilate glucose for energy, leaving you feeling mentally and physically exhausted.

Similarly, when there isn't enough insulin to help your body and brain utilize glucose, you begin to break down muscle and stored fat in an attempt to provide fuel to hungry cells.

Blood sugar imbalances can interfere with your neurotransmitters, like your happiness hormone serotonin, contributing to symptoms of depression. Insulin resistance also throws your pleasure-and-reward neurotransmitter dopamine off-balance; this can trigger low-dopamine feelings of hopelessness, worthlessness, or feeling unmotivated and short-tempered.

Insulin resistance is also a key issue in weight loss. When your cells aren't able to receive energy from glucose, they rely on fat stores instead. Your body literally will not allow you to lose weight, since it needs to preserve the fat for energy. No amount of reduced calories will help you to lose weight, until your cells begin to accept the insulin again.

Insulin Resistance in Your Brain

New research suggests that insulin resistance begins in the brain. Insulin receptors have been detected in the brain, independent of the insulin circulating in your body. This "brain insulin" is now believed to have a significant impact on your brain function, metabolism, and body weight.

When your brain cannot use insulin properly, too much sugar stays in the bloodstream, damaging the brain's tissue and circulatory system. This brain insulin resistance contributes to weight gain and even degenerative brain diseases, because excess insulin reduces your brain's ability to clear out amyloid plaques that contribute to Alzheimer's disease.

Your hypothalamus regulates the amount of insulin in your body and brain, constantly monitoring blood levels of insulin and signaling your pancreas to produce more or less insulin, based on the amount in your bloodstream. Your hypothalamus also serves as the satiety center of your brain, controlling hunger and food intake. Insulin regulates your appetite through your hypothalamus, so brain insulin resistance results in increased food intake and weight gain. It can also contribute to metabolic diseases like diabetes, mood disorders, and neuro-degenerative diseases like Parkinson's and Alzheimer's.

BRAIN INSULIN AND YOUR HEALTH

Insulin resistance in the brain can contribute to a myriad of health challenges.

Weight. Insulin resistance in the brain contributes to obesity. Healthy insulin levels in your brain reduce hunger and boost your metabolic rate. Research has found that infusing insulin directly into the brains of animals reduced their appetites by affecting the levels of various hormones that control hunger.

Temperature. Insulin resistance in the brain decreases thermogenesis (burning energy to keep your body temperature up), which lowers your metabolic rate.

Cognitive function. Insulin plays a key role in cognitive processing and forming memories; this is the reason why diabetics experience memory and cognition issues. Interestingly, Alzheimer's disease is often referred to as type 3 diabetes.

Inflammation. The buildup of extra insulin (from insulin resistance) increases C-reactive proteins (linked to brain inflammation) and the buildup of amyloid plaques (correlated with Alzheimer's disease).

Mood disorders. Low insulin levels impact your brain's "feel good" neurotransmitters, like dopamine and serotonin, and increase brain inflammation, both of which play a pivotal role in depression. Research on intranasal insulin correlated enhanced brain insulin function with enhanced mood, increased self-confidence, reduced anger, and improved executive function.

Hormone balance. Insulin surges increase testosterone production. High testosterone blunts cells' insulin receptor sites, leading to a vicious cycle of insulin resistance and hormonal imbalance. High testosterone in women impacts levels of estrogen and progesterone, affecting motivation, drive, and mood. In men, insulin resistance promotes excess estrogen that may lead to excess tissue in breasts and hips.

OLFACTORY DELIVERY OF INSULIN TO THE BRAIN

Because the sense of smell is the most expedient channel into the brain, essential oils are an ideal remedy to balance blood sugar within the brain.

Insulin receptors are located on nerve cells throughout your brain, with the highest density concentrated in your olfactory bulb. Intranasal insulin (inhaling insulin)—a non-invasive method of insulin delivery—increases insulin levels in your brain to overcome brain insulin resistance and improve brain function. Because the olfactory nerves evolved before the brain, they are not protected by the blood-brain barrier. This is why the olfactory channel is used in anesthesia, because it is the most direct route into the brain. This means that inhaling intranasal insulin or essential oils with insulin-enhancing properties can help increase brain insulin and brain function. Essential oils, when inhaled, deliver the appropriate remedy straight into specific areas of your brain.

UNBLOCK INSULIN RECEPTORS USING ESSENTIAL OILS

Essential oils may help clean your insulin receptors to restore proper insulin signaling. There is evidence that phenylpropanoid, a component found in the essential oils of cassia, cinnamon, clove, and tarragon, can bind with cell receptors and consequently inhibit or activate your cell receptors to help brain cells better respond to the presence of insulin. Eugenol, an active constituent in clove oil, has been shown to interact with cell receptors and inhibit or activate signaling cascades; this is how it effectively inhibits symptoms of pain and inflammation. New research is finding that essential oils like oregano and myrtle when inhaled or topically applied might help support healthy blood sugar levels by enhancing the function of digestive enzymes.

Cinnamon Helps Sensitize Insulin Receptors

Research published in the *Journal of Diabetes Science and Technology* finds that "components of cinnamon make insulin more efficient." More specifically, a liquid extract of cinnamon (like those included in cinnamon and cassia essential oils) increases insulin sensitivity and reduces insulin resistance.

"Liquid herbs work faster and better in most patients—anywhere from two to ten times faster and better than any dried herbs or tablet," according to endocrinology specialist Janet Lang. Research backs this up, noting that "when compared to herbs, spices, and medicinal extracts for insulin-like or insulin-potentiating activity, cinnamon extracts potentiated insulin activity more than twentyfold, higher than any other compound tested at comparable dilutions."

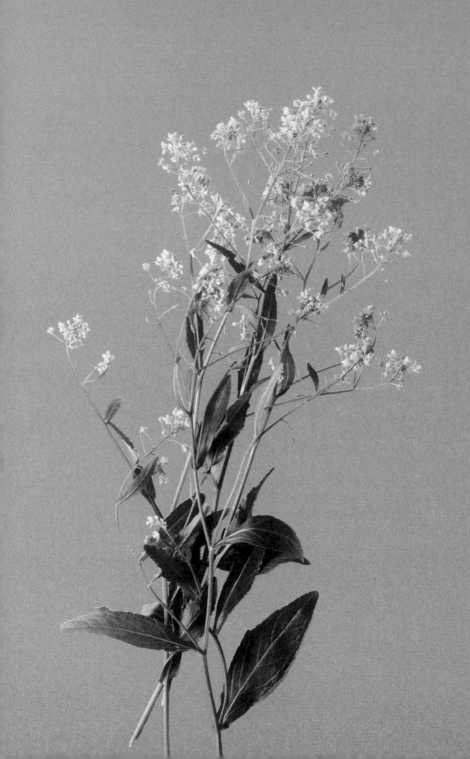

Stimulating Your Brain
and Improving Focus

Now that you understand the important roles that circulation and blood sugar play in optimizing your brain health, let's move on to how you can strategically stimulate mechanisms in your brain to help you improve your focus and mental energy throughout your day. Whether you have a major work presentation to write or a day of juggling errands, you need your mind to be in top form—and that's where brain-boosting essential oils can quickly come to your rescue.

Your Prefontal Cortex

Your ability to sustain focus is driven by your prefrontal cortex. This is the part of your frontal lobe that's located in the front portion of the brain, behind your forehead—and its job is an important one. The circuitry in your frontal lobe helps your brain sort through stimulation to decide what information is relevant and what needs to be ignored. This helps you regulate movements, control impulses, use language, focus attention, make decisions, and correct errors.

This ability to inhibit certain behaviors helps your brain focus on important tasks, improving your thinking and processing speed. The prefrontal cortex is responsible for executive functioning, which includes thinking, organizing, problem solving, memory, concentration, and decision making. Without your prefrontal cortex, you would have trouble finishing a book, remembering to pay your bills, or returning phone calls.

What's more, a decrease in this lobe's function often lies at the root of mood issues like depression and behavioral problems such as ADD and ADHD. Depression is actually considered a frontal lobe impairment. Research shows that decreased firing of messages from the frontal lobe results in lower levels of motivation and a decreased sense of well-being. This helps to explain why when most people get depressed, they also have a hard time concentrating, focusing, and remembering details.

A healthy frontal lobe, on the other hand, allows you to reason and suppress impulses. Children with ADHD demonstrate delays in frontal cortex development that correlates with an inability to suppress immediate desires and impulses. Think about how a young child might shout out an answer without waiting for the teacher to call on him. Kids with ADHD lack inhibition and have decreased activation in their frontal lobes compared to those without the diagnosis, according to research from McGill University. Similar brain-imaging studies found the prefrontal cortex in individuals diagnosed with ADHD to be smaller than that of individuals without the diagnosis.

Your prefrontal cortex also helps calm your stress response by chemically moderating or inhibiting signals from the threat alert center of your brain known as your amygdala. When this prefrontal-amygdala connection is weak, excessive anxiety can result.

When you activate your prefrontal cortex, you enhance your brain's ability to plan, organize, and see the big picture. When the prefrontal cortex is not firing on all cylinders, it loses processing speed and deficits of inhibition and focus can occur, resulting in poor internal supervision, short attention span, distractibility, disorganization, hyperactivity, impulse control problems, difficulty learning from past errors, a lack of forethought, and procrastination. Strengthening the prefrontal cortex also exerts a moderating influence on the more impulsive and less flexible structures of your limbic system, helping you calm repetitive thought patterns and anxiety.

HOW POOR IS YOUR FOCUS?

You'll want to keep an eye out for clues that your prefrontal cortex isn't firing at its best so that you can give it the essential oil tune-up it needs. Are you feeling:

- Easily distracted? You become easily preoccupied by your phone or social media.
- Mentally wiped? It's difficult to concentrate for long periods of time, such as on long drives or during continuous mental tasks.
- Unable to sustain your attention? It's challenging to pay attention in school, at meetings, or during long conversations.
- Impulsive? You have a hard time restraining yourself and controlling impulses or desires. You may say things before thinking about the consequences.
- Argumentative? You might seek out conflict to stimulate an underactive prefrontal cortex.

- Depressed? You feel moody. That's because when the prefrontal cortex is underactive, it can't moderate the emotional limbic area of your brain.
- Disorganized? Your home, work environment, car, and closet are a cluttered mess. A common sign of an underactive prefrontal cortex is disorganized, unfinished paperwork.
- Unable to let go? You may repeat events or thoughts or struggle to get a song out of your head.
- Lack of motivation? You may have low interest, drive, or enthusiasm for getting things done or struggle to start tasks in the first place.
- Unable to finish tasks? You may start a project and move on to the next before completing it. You get bored easily.
- Trouble listening? You lack the sustained attention required to listen to the person speaking. This contributes to a lack of empathy.
- All over the place, in general? This is a sign of poor executive function. An underactive prefrontal cortex contributes to an inability to organize, sequence, or plan projects and to oversee the details of a situation or conversation, while maintaining a vision of the whole. You might also struggle with analytical thoughts or have a hard time making decisions.

HOW THE BRAIN LOSES THE ABILITY TO FOCUS

Chronic stress has the ability to flip a switch that inhibits connections to the prefrontal cortex, which lays down durable scaffolding linked to anxiety, depression, and post–traumatic stress disorder (PTSD). Similarly, modern technology scatters your attention and weakens the brain's wiring for focus. Just like a muscle atrophies from being underused, your prefrontal cortex shrinks with lack of focus. Your brain is "use it or lose it": if the prefrontal cortex is neglected, it begins to atrophy. As a result, the degraded brain wiring can no longer focus, be attentive, organize, or build sequences and ideas.

When connections to the prefrontal cortex are inhibited, you need to reactivate these connections to turn down stress. You can manually stimulate them by topically applying essential oils, such as peppermint, rosemary, or the Focus Blend (see page 186), on reflex points on the forehead, like your temples. Stimulating your prefrontal cortex (through thought patterns, essential oils, or a combination of both) can prime it to develop new brain pathways.

ESSENTIAL OILS OFFER THE MOST DIRECT PATH
TO YOUR FRONTAL LOBE

Your olfactory nerve travels directly to your frontal lobe through a bone known as the cribriform plate at the top of your sinuses. Smell is the only sense that does not travel to the thalamus (the relay center for all sensory signals) before accessing the forebrain. All other senses send signals through the thalamus first, which then sends the signals to the proper areas of the brain for perception.

Your nostrils travel to separate sides of the brain. More specifically, your right nostril corresponds to the right side of the brain, and the left nostril to the left side, allowing you to target specific areas of each side of your brain differently.

Panic Attack Hack

Anxiety can be triggered by overactivity and dominance of the right frontal lobe of your brain. The right brain processes the emotional aspects of the human experience, giving you empathy and compassion, but in overdrive, the right brain can contribute to heightened emotions and anxiety.

Functional neurologist Dr. Titus Chiu suggests strategically inhaling essential oils, like lavender or orange, through your left nostril to activate your left frontal lobe and balance the over-activity of the right frontal lobe. This creates balance between the left and right hemispheres of the brain, which then leads to feelings of calm and helps halt panic attacks.

BALANCING YOUR BRAIN'S HEMISPHERES

Direct access from the nostrils to the different sides of your brain allows you to topically apply essential oils to stimulate and balance the following imbalances in different hemispheres of your brain.

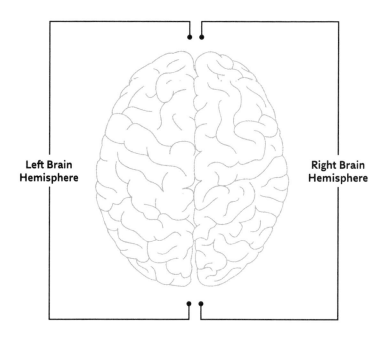

Left Brain Hemisphere

Right Brain Hemisphere

The signs of left brain imbalance include:

- Poor math skills
- Poor verbal skills
- Poor reading and spelling skills
- Fine-motor problems
- Poor auditory processing
- Weak immune response
- Poor memory for details
- Misses small details
- Poor self-esteem
- Poor motivation
- Task avoidance

The signs of right brain imbalance include:

- Awkward/clumsy
- Hyperactive/anxious
- Poor nonverbal skills
- Impulsive/lacks focus
- Lacks emotional control
- Obsessive/repetitive behaviors
- Immature social behavior
- Allergies/autoimmunity
- Disinterest in physical activities
- Misses the big picture
- Poor eye contact
- Unaware of body space

Blood Flow and Concentration

When you concentrate, blood flow increases in your brain, especially in your prefrontal cortex. This increased blood flow allows you to focus, stay on task, and think ahead. Research has found that blood flow actually decreases when people diagnosed with ADD and ADHD try to concentrate, making it harder to stay focused.

The brains of those with ADD and ADHD also have low levels of the excitatory neurotransmitter norepinephrine, which helps the brain and body mobilize for action, along with dopamine, which helps control the brain's reward and pleasure center. Medications used to treat ADHD often help improve the level of activation of the prefrontal cortex by enhancing the levels of dopamine and norepinephrine.

AMYGDALA HIJACK

Your amygdala identifies potential danger and triggers your initial automatic, emotional reaction. Then your prefrontal cortex—your brain's decision center—assesses the situation before driving you to act. It collaborates with your amygdala fear center to help interpret and balance your response to potential dangers.

For example, if you are hiking in the woods and think you see a snake on the ground, your amygdala might trigger an immediate response, causing you to physically jump back. It then alerts your prefrontal cortex to assess the situation. If your prefrontal cortex determines that the snake is actually a stick, your amygdala calms down as does your fear response.

As long as the connection between your prefrontal cortex and your amygdala remains strong, your fear response can remain in check. Chronic stress can shift this balance—speeding the flow of electrical signals to your amygdala fear center and weakening the connection to your inhibitory prefrontal cortex. This poor connection, known as amygdala hijack, shuts down your ability to calm stress and sets the stage for anxiety, depression, and other limbic system imbalances.

Similarly, if your frontal cortex is damaged or understimulated, planning the slightest task is very difficult, if not impossible, and anxiety is common. Functional brain imaging clearly illustrates how engaging your prefrontal cortex helps regulate and calm amygdala reactivity and control of emotion-related behavior. When not kept in check by the prefrontal cortex, exaggerated amygdala reactivity can present as depression, anxiety, impulsive aggression, and personality disorders. These symptoms are also common among individuals recovering from a frontal lobe injury.

Frequent stimulation of your prefrontal cortex supports a healthy connection to your amygdala, which helps to calm your response to fear stimulus and also to unravel and heal conditioned fear responses, like anxiety and post–traumatic stress disorder (PTSD).

THE PREFRONTAL CORTEX AND ADD/ADHD AND DEPRESSION

A poor connection between your right or left prefrontal cortex and your amygdala also can present as ADD/ADHD symptoms. For example, if your left prefrontal cortex is underactive during concentration while your amygdala is overactive, it can present as brain dysregulation, ADD/ADHD, and symptoms of depression such as moodiness, irritability, low self-esteem, negative thought loops, decreased interest in activities previously considered fun, feelings of hopelessness, and a tendency for social isolation. This is because your amygdala sets your emotional tone, controlling how happy or sad you are, affecting your motivation, drive, attention, and ability to connect emotionally with others.

Strengthening the left prefrontal cortex by topically applying a stimulatory essential oil like peppermint or rosemary over your left temple or inhaling through your left nostril may stimulate the function of your prefrontal cortex to exert a moderating influence on the more impulsive and less flexible structures of your amygdala.

STIMULATE THE PREFRONTAL CORTEX WITH ESSENTIAL OILS

Topically applying essential oils to reflex points on your forehead can help increase blood flow to the area and strengthen your prefrontal cortex. This, in turn, helps improve brain function, focus, memory, and processing speed. It also helps prevent and reverse cognitive decline.

These reflex points develop in vitro to support circulation in a developing fetus, while the heart develops. These circuits remain even after the heart fully develops to support circulation and activate blood flow to specific organs or regions of the brain.

When we are under stress, blood goes to the back of our brains, where long-term memories are stored. Placing appropriate essential oils over these points on the forehead helps shift the energy and blood flow from the more emotional midbrain areas to the prefrontal cortex, which prompts a calmer mind and rational, logical thinking. Research finds that these neurovascular points switch off, like a circuit breaker, in response to stress. Applying essential oils to these points switches them back on, increasing blood flow to the prefrontal cortex.

Stimulating the reflex points on the inside of the eyebrows, over the temples, and at the base of the hairline on both the right and left sides of the forehead increases blood flow to the area. Essential oils, like black pepper, also increase blood flow to targeted regions of the brain. The combination of specific oils in the Focus Blend (see page 186) on specific reflex points amplifies stimulation to that region of the brain.

The hands can also be used to stimulate the forehead points. Research indicates that the longer you hold the points, the more the stress will fade. Applying essential oils to the points allows you to hold the energy for significantly longer, resulting in greater health improvements.

Many practitioners find that these forehead points often test better than the organ points or the ears for oil application. This technique has been successfully integrated in combination with clinical techniques like the Five Element Meridian Release and the Emotional Stress Release taught in Touch for Health, a popular system for balancing posture, attitude, and energy to relieve stress and pain.

IMPROVE ADD/ADHD SYMPTOMS WITH ESSENTIAL OILS

Natural remedies like essential oils may improve ADD/ADHD symptoms, according to the late Dr. Terry Friedmann. A blend of cedarwood, frankincense, lavender, and vetiver (see Essential Oils for ADD and ADHD on page 201) was found to be particularly beneficial for children with ADD/ADHD. When children with ADD/ADHD inhaled the essential oil blend three times a day for thirty days, they demonstrated improved focus and calmer behavior. The inhalation of the oils also improved brain wave patterns as measured via an electro-encephalograph device, which measures electrical impulses moving through the brain. Researchers observed that the essential oil blends shifted brain waves from the lack-of-focus theta state into the alert beta state. Improvements in beta-theta ratios were noted following the use of vetiver essential oil. Parents similarly noted improvements in behavior at home and performance at school.

FOREHEAD APPLICATION POINTS

Meridians are energy pathways in the body that nourish, maintain, and support your organ systems. Traditional Chinese Medicine (TCM) works to remove any blockages in the meridian system (either with acupuncture needles or essential oils) to prevent energy deficiencies or surpluses that contribute to health imbalances.

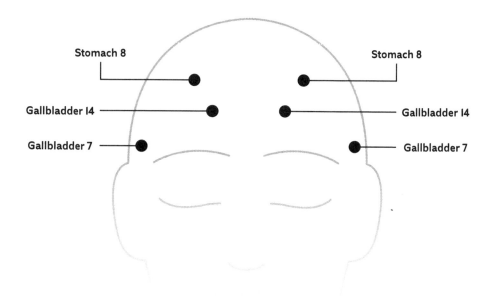

Stomach 8: Located near the hairline at the corner of the forehead. Oils applied on this point are known to relieve pain and dizziness, including vertigo. This is an especially good point for alleviating headache and migraine pain.

Gallbladder 14: Located on the forehead, directly above the center of your eye, one finger's width above your eyebrows in the depression on the superciliary arch. Known as the mental healing point, oils applied on this point help to improve memory and recall, transform negative thoughts, reprogram your mind, and release mental stress.

Gallbladder 7: Located on the sides of the face at the point of depression of the lower temples, a half inch outside the eyebrows. Oils applied on this point improves memory and concentration and enhances mental state. This application point also helps reduce dizziness and headaches.

REDUCING STRESS, IMPROVING MOOD, AND LOSING WEIGHT

It takes a lot of energy to heal. Stress, emotional upset, and extra weight can drain your physical and emotional energy. If your brain is stuck in a chronic stress pattern and believes survival is at risk, it will channel all available energy and resources that could be used for healing toward survival. This will impact your mood, leading to depression and anxiety, and impact your weight. Essential oils can help your brain to shift out of a stress response, freeing up energy and resources that your body can then use to heal, feel happier, and drop extra pounds.

Reducing Stress

Stress is the root of all disease. It shuts down digestion, detoxification, and immune function. It contributes to systemic inflammation, which can impact your gut and your mood, throwing blood sugar levels out of balance and contributing to sleep issues and fatigue. And stress hormones, such as cortisol, are corrosive to the body and brain.

Stress is your reaction to real or perceived potentially dangerous situations. We often think of stress in terms of psychological challenges, like a stressful job, relationship, or situation. While those are clearly stressful to the body, they are not the only source of stress. A stressor can be any physical, environmental, physiological, emotional, or psychological stimulus that the mind perceives as a threat. Your stress response supplies you with the energy you need to survive.

> **Physical stress.** Anything stressing the body—including physical injuries, headache, chronic inflammation, pain, scars or surgeries, structural misalignment like a clenched jaw, or even physical exercise—can stress your system.
>
> **Environmental stress.** Toxins in the environment—including mold, pesticides, herbicides, pollution, chemicals in the home (skin-care and cleaning products), chlorine or fluoride in tap water, food additives or preservatives, electromagnetic emissions from cell phones, Wi-Fi, computers, cell towers, or smart meters—can add to your stress load.
>
> **Physiological stress.** Even natural bodily processes can contribute to stress levels. For example, any low-level infection; parasites; fever; food sensitivity; blood sugar imbalance; vitamin or mineral deficiency; imbalance in gut flora; leaky gut; constipation; sleep deficiency;

dehydration; digestive, cardiovascular, or skin issues; autoimmunity; liver toxicity; or kidney stress add to the cumulative stress level.

Psychological or external emotional stress. Experiences like the death of a loved one, divorce, surgery, financial hardship, unhealthy relationship or work environment, and other conditions that provoke feelings of helplessness can increase stress.

Internal emotional stress. Your body cannot differentiate a perceived emotional or anticipatory thought-driven threat from an actual physical stress. Your body mobilizes a stress response to thoughts of fear, anger, and grief; thought patterns of guilt or jealousy; and feelings such as a lack of control, poor boundaries, self-abuse, shame, humiliation, unworthiness, betrayal, shock, and trauma.

The Interplay Between Stressors

Stresses are additive and cumulative. The volume of stresses, the intensity of each stress, and the frequency and duration of time combine to form a total stress load. The more you layer on, the more likely you are to overwhelm your system. Imagine a cup of water that is completely full. Even an additional drop of water will cause the cup to overflow. Stress in the body is like that—when our stress bucket is full, it easily overflows.

Every stressor you remove expands your resilience. Even tidying your environment and purging items that you no longer need or use can be a powerful stress reliever.

The physiological stress from the process of running the body accounts for at least 30 percent of your body's total stress load. When attempting to reduce your stress load, it's important to balance these physiological functions.

Imbalances in blood sugar can trigger a cortisol response and increase stress. An inflamed gut can become leaky, whereby harmful substances like toxins or pathogens leak through the gut lining into the bloodstream and put physiological stress on the body. Malabsorption of nutrients depletes the body of the vitamins and minerals necessary to chemically support the stress response. When toxins aren't removed from the body, they recirculate and become a stressor.

The Duration of Stress

Short-term stress is a normal part of life, keeping us alert, motivated, and able to avoid danger. You are designed to experience stress, react to it, then return to balance. It is the chronic or ongoing, prolonged physical, mental, and emotional stress that fuels chronic inflammation and depresses your immune system. Chronic stress triggers physical symptoms like elevated blood pressure, stomach ulcers, pain, fatigue, and headaches, along with emotional responses like anxiety, depression, panic attacks, and irritability.

Stress Impacts Three Regions of Your Brain

Stress triggers a domino effect in the body to go on high alert, evoking a fight-or-flight response and freeing up all available energy and resources to escape the perceived threat. This is known as a stress response, and it impacts the following three regions of the brain: the sympathetic nervous system, the hypothalamic-pituitary-adrenal (HPA) axis, and the limbic system.

SYMPATHETIC NERVOUS SYSTEM
Your body's first line of defense against stress is the sympathetic branch of your autonomic nervous system (see page 25). Stress activates your survival response, releasing hormones like adrenaline and routing blood flow away from your brain toward your heart, lungs, and limbs to help you flee from danger.

HPA AXIS STRESS RESPONSE
Stress mobilizes energy in the form of the stress hormones, released through a complex hormonal cascade in your endocrine system, involving a three-part chain of command, known as the HPA axis (see page 108). These HPA interactions continue until your hormones reach the levels that your body needs, and then a series of chemical reactions begin to switch them off.

LIMBIC SYSTEM
Your limbic system is the emotional center of your brain, composed of a complex system of nerves and networks that serve as a key safety filter, analyzing and filtering incoming stimuli—including feelings of fear, anger, grief, despair, or hopelessness—to determine whether they are a threat to your survival.

THE HYPOTHALAMIC-PITUITARY-ADRENAL (HPA) AXIS

H Hypothalamus, a pearl-size region of the brain that serves as the control center for neural and hormonal messages received from or sent to the body. Upon receiving a stress message, your hypothalamus releases a corticotrophin-releasing hormone (CRH) to signal your pituitary gland.

P Pituitary, your hormonal middle man, which receives hormonal messages from the hypothalamus and translates these messages into hormones distributed to the thyroid, adrenals, and sex organs. When triggered by the hypothalamus, the pituitary sends a message to your adrenals to produce cortisol.

A Adrenal glands produce and release the stress hormone cortisol. Cortisol's main job is to provide energy to fuel your body through a stressful situation. For example, cortisol raises the sugar in your bloodstream to increase the energy available for a stress response. Chronic cortisol release keeps your body's repair and healing processes shut down.

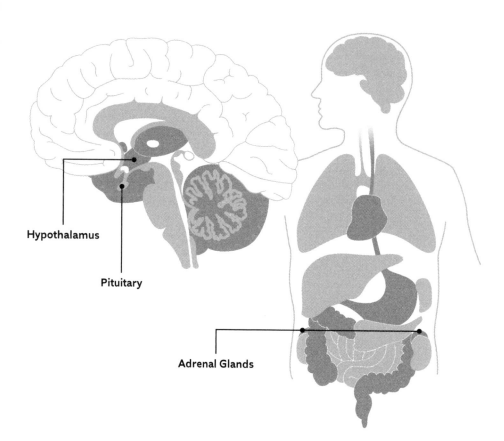

Hypothalamus

Pituitary

Adrenal Glands

The Hypothalamus

Your hypothalamus oversees your body's stress response by continuously monitoring your blood levels for cortisol and adjusting the resulting signals sent to the body to either produce more or less cortisol. (See page 125 for more information on the imbalances in the hypothalamus and pituitary.)

When your hypothalamus gets the signal that the right volume of cortisol has been released, it inhibits the signals to produce more cortisol. This is known as a negative feedback loop that works only when accurate feedback is received by your hypothalamus. Chronic and prolonged stress can overstimulate your hypothalamus and compromise its ability to receive clear signals. This can cause the hypothalamus to continue signaling your adrenals to release excessive cortisol. The ongoing release of cortisol then hard-wires stress pathways in your brain, predisposing you to more stress and symptoms like anxiety, depression, post–traumatic stress disorder (PTSD), and other mood disorders.

The healthy function of your hypothalamus determines the healthy function of your adrenals and your ability to manage stress. Essential oils can help reboot the hypothalamus to restore healthy function (see Hypothalamus Blend on page 184).

The Pituitary Gland

If the hypothalamus is your CEO, your pituitary functions more like your chief operating officer. Responding to hormonal and nerve signals from the hypothalamus, the pituitary gland sends hormonal messages to other endocrine glands, directing them to stimulate or inhibit the release of their respective hormones, thus regulating various physiological processes, including stress, growth, reproduction, lactation, thyroid function, and water metabolism.

To help boost pituitary gland health, use frankincense essential oil from Somalia, which is strongly anti-inflammatory. Apply a small dab to the middle of your forehead or to the roof of your mouth up to five times daily.

The Adrenal Glands

Your adrenals are small triangular-shaped glands that sit on top of your kidneys and support your body's response to stress by secreting the hormones cortisol and adrenaline that help you mobilize resources—increasing energy, heart rate, and muscle tone—to improve your chances of survival. They direct all available energy either to fighting the stressor or fleeing from it, and they depress everything not critical to immediate survival, like immune function and your ability to digest, detoxify, and reproduce.

Cortisol has a dualistic relationship with inflammation—meaning it can be both pro- and anti-inflammatory, and the dynamic evolves over time. In the short term, cortisol calms inflammation to enhance your chances of survival. Over time, chronically high cortisol levels decrease the sensitivity of your tissues to cortisol, undermining its effectiveness in calming inflammation.

ADRENAL RESILIENCE

Every stress response triggers an adrenal response, so maintaining the health and resilience of your adrenals will help boost energy levels and your tolerance to stress. When your adrenals are dealing with a lot of stress, they either overfunction or underfunction.

If your adrenals are overfunctioning, they slip into overdrive, a condition known as hyper-cortisol, which produces symptoms such as:

——— A tendency to be a "night person"
——— Difficulty falling asleep
——— A tendency to be keyed up and to have trouble calming down
——— Blood pressure above 120/80
——— Feeling wired or jittery after drinking coffee
——— Clenching or grinding teeth
——— Calm on the outside, troubled on the inside
——— Arthritic tendencies
——— Perspire easily
——— Tendency to sprain ankles or to get shin splints

If they are underfunctioning, they become so depleted that you are unable to release or produce the hormones to react to a stressful situation, commonly referred to as adrenal fatigue, which produces symptoms like:

——— Being a slow starter in the morning
——— Fatigue not relieved by sleep
——— Chronic lower back pain that is worse with fatigue
——— Becoming dizzy when standing up suddenly
——— Pain after or difficulty maintaining chiropractic correction
——— Craving salty foods or oversalting foods before tasting
——— Afternoon yawning or headache
——— A need to wear sunglasses even when it is not bright

Different supplements are often recommended for hyper versus fatigued adrenals, but the main goal is to return the adrenals to balance. Essential oils can play a key role here.

SUPPORT ADRENAL BALANCE WITH ESSENTIAL OILS
Essential oils can be used like adaptogenic herbs—which help the body adapt to stress—to support the adrenal glands for the optimal energy reserves required for healing. Plants and essential oils are homeostatic, meaning they do not force change on the body but simply balance out what your body needs, either stimulating or inhibiting chemical messengers to help return your system to balance.

This is especially helpful for your adrenal glands, which can toggle between overfunction and underfunction several times a day. If you were to test cortisol levels over a twenty-four-hour cycle, you might notice that at times they are too high and at other times too low. Unlike supplements that either stimulate or calm cortisol levels, essential oils meet your body where it's at and provide balance (see page 183 for recommended essential oils for adrenal balance).

Limbic System

You might think of the limbic system as a highly sensitized security system. It categorizes all sensory input as either a threat or a nonthreat, based on past experience. Your limbic system includes your amygdala (associated with emotions), hypothalamus (regulates autonomic nervous system and hormones), and cingulate gyrus (regulates blood pressure, heart rate, and attention). The limbic system also impacts long-term memory through the hippocampus, the area of the brain at play during those emotions or memories triggered by a particular smell.

If your limbic system is damaged from chemical exposure, toxic molds, viruses, infections, inflammation, trauma, or stress, this filtering process can become impaired and alter the way that the brain and body interpret, encode, and react to sensory or emotional stimuli that they would usually disregard as not representing a danger to the body.

When not functioning properly, a hypersensitive limbic system categorizes nonthreatening stimuli as threatening, triggering involuntary trauma patterns and contributing to distorted unconscious reactions, sensory perceptions, and protective responses. Over time, this state of hyper-arousal can weaken other systems in your body and negatively impact your ability to rest, digest, detoxify, heal, stabilize your mood, and maintain motor and cognitive function.

In other words, limbic system impairment can sensitize your brain to a negative stress response that leads to chronic sickness behavior and conditions like chronic fatigue, fibromyalgia, and multiple chemical sensitivity.

THE SYMPTOMS OF LIMBIC SYSTEM IMPAIRMENT

Some indications that your limbic system function could be improved include:

—— Brain fog, or an inability to concentrate or focus
—— Low energy and fatigue
—— Chronic joint and/or muscle pain
—— Heightened sensory perceptions, including smell, taste, light, sound, or electromagnetic sensitivities
—— Sensitivity to perfumes, household cleaners, personal hygiene products, or other chemicals
—— Anxiety, worry, mood swings, or panic attacks
—— Depression
—— Sleep-related issues
—— Food sensitivities
—— Headaches
—— Dwelling on past negative events or expecting negative outcomes
—— Short-term memory problems

HEAL THE LIMBIC SYSTEM WITH ESSENTIAL OILS

Essential oils can be used to help rewire your brain to reduce stress by interrupting thought patterns and emotions that trigger a stress response and resetting the volume on your limbic system's threat perception, so that it no longer fires too rapidly or too often. Rewiring the neural circuits in your limbic system can help strengthen your emotional resilience and calm your response to stress, pain, fatigue, and unpleasant emotional thoughts and experiences.

The sense of smell links directly to the amygdala in the limbic lobe of the brain, which stores and releases memories of emotional trauma. Smell has a direct route to the limbic system, since it is physically located near the olfactory bulb and can often mobilize long-forgotten memories and emotions that can help rewire neural circuits and calm the overfiring of your danger signal. Essential oils, with their ability to directly access areas of the brain associated with emotions and memory, are uniquely suited to help you reset threat perception and help to calm the overfiring of protective mechanisms that either fire too rapidly or too often (see Parasympathetic Blend, page 169).

The Connection Between Smell and Emotions

In 1989, Dr. Joseph LeDoux, a professor of science at New York University and director of the Emotional Brain Institute, discovered that the amygdala plays a much more critical role in the storage and release of memories of emotional traumas than had been previously believed. Dr. LeDoux's research was the first to recognize that the amygdala triggers an emotional reaction before the thinking brain has fully processed nerve signals. In other words, emotional reactions and memories can be formed *and released* without any conscious, cognitive participation.

Olfactory researcher Rachel Herz built upon this understanding of how the brain processes emotion, noting in a *Scientific American* article entitled "Do Scents Affect People's Moods or Work Performance?" that "the olfactory bulbs are part of the limbic system and directly connect with limbic structures that process emotion (the amygdala) and associative learning (the hippocampus). No other sensory system has this type of intimate link with the neural areas of emotion and associative learning; therefore, there is a strong neurological basis for why odors trigger emotional connections." Herz also wrote, "The emotional power of smell-triggered memory has an intensity unequaled by sight- and sound-triggered ones." Since sound is not as effective as smell for releasing memory trauma, talking about your problems might not heal the underlying emotions as effectively as releasing them through the use of aromatic essential oils.

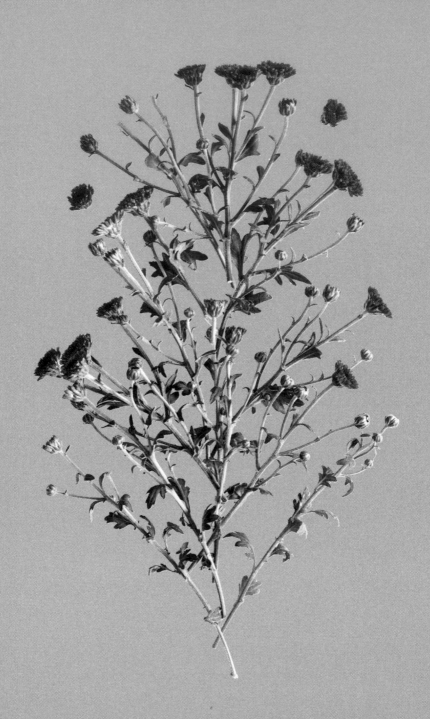

Improving Mood

Neurotransmitters are chemical messengers that carry information in the form of electric signals between the cells in your body and the brain. Your brain functions best when messages get delivered quickly and easily. When the strength and speed of neurotransmitter signals are compromised, it impacts how you feel and function, influencing your mood, memory, learning, self-esteem, anxiety levels, and motivation.

Neurotransmitters

The brain uses neurotransmitters to regulate critical functions in your body, including breathing, heart rate, muscle movement, appetite, digestion, mood and concentration, and sleep cycles.

A neurotransmitter is released from the surface of one brain cell into an extracellular space, which forms part of the synapse—the connecting space between two brain cells. Once released into the synapse, the neurotransmitter travels across the extracellular space and binds to specific proteins—called cell receptors—located on the surface of the receiving brain cell. When the neurotransmitter binds to these receptors, it sets up a cascade of chemical reactions within the receiving cell to carry the electrical signal through that cell and farther into your brain.

Pharmaceutical drugs use the same pathways to support emotional and psychological concerns like anxiety and depression. Drugs like barbiturates, anesthetics, benzodiazepines, antidepressants, and anti-seizure medications bind to cell receptors in your brain to help enhance your mood.

NEUROTRANSMITTERS

The brain uses neurotransmitters to regulate critical functions in your body.

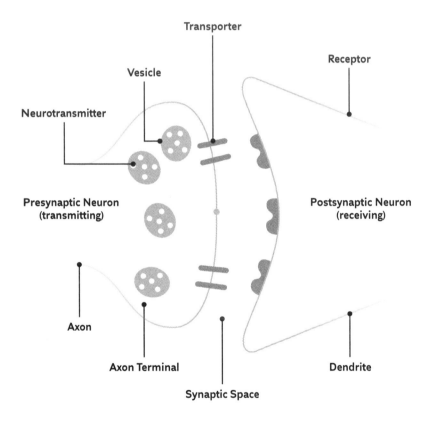

Transporter

Receptor

Vesicle

Neurotransmitter

Presynaptic Neuron
(transmitting)

Postsynaptic Neuron
(receiving)

Axon

Axon Terminal

Dendrite

Synaptic Space

HOW ESSENTIAL OILS IMPACT NEUROTRANSMITTERS

Essential oils work in the same way to stimulate your neurotransmitters. When you inhale an essential oil, it sends a signal to your olfactory system and tells the brain to call on the appropriate neurotransmitters, like mood-regulating serotonin and dopamine. Certain essential oils, like lavender, can bind to the receptors on your cells that receive your body's calming neurotransmitter, GABA (gamma-aminobutyric acid), to help balance your brain's level of excitation and inhibition that is vital for normal brain function and a healthy nervous system. In addition, linalool, an active ingredient of lavender oil, has been shown to modulate the transmission of GABA in your brain by activating GABA receptors and blocking brain signals that activate your stress response. This calms your nervous system.

Some supplements, like 5-hydroxytryptophan (5-HTP), and nutrients in foods, such as choline, can influence the production of neurotransmitters. Tryptophan is the amino acid precursor, or building block, of serotonin. Remedies must be able to cross the blood-brain barrier to modify your brain's neurotransmitter response. Neurotransmitters like dopamine and serotonin lack the necessary transport mechanisms to cross the blood-brain barrier, while lipid-soluble molecules do not.

INHIBITORY OR EXCITATORY NEUROTRANSMITTERS

Inhibitory neurotransmitters *decrease* the action of a nerve impulse, whereas excitatory neurotransmitters *increase* the action. You can stimulate an excitatory neurotransmitter for more energy and focus or stimulate an inhibitory neurotransmitter to calm your system.

Many of the drugs designed to support your mood and brain function work on this principle, altering the balance of different neurotransmitters in your brain or compensating for an imbalance by either enhancing the effects of the neurotransmitter or preventing their reuptake. Beta-blocker drugs work by blocking neurotransmitter receptors. You've probably heard of selective serotonin reuptake inhibitors (SSRIs), a class of drugs often used as antidepressants that work by limiting how cells reabsorb the neurotransmitter serotonin and how it binds to receptors.

Essential oils work in a similar fashion, by activating or inhibiting excitatory and inhibitory neurotransmitters. Inhaling the appropriate essential oils can communicate signals to the olfactory system and stimulate the brain to release neurotransmitters that help regulate your mood. For example, research explained in an article in *Current Drug Targets* entitled "Aromatherapy and the Central Nerve System" found that smelling bergamot, lavender, and lemon essential oils help to trigger your brain to release serotonin and dopamine.

A blend of basil, cardamom, holy basil, peppermint, and rosemary can calm the excitatory neurotransmitter noradrenaline (see Focus Blend on page 186). Ylang-ylang stimulates the release of endorphins.

BALANCE NEUROTRANSMITTERS WITH ESSENTIAL OILS

Essential oils can help bring your neurotransmitters back into balance, supplementing deficiencies and calming excesses, which can help you naturally balance your mood. They can bind to cell receptor sites and block, activate, or modulate the impact of neurotransmitters.

Adrenaline (Epinephrine)

The excitatory neurotransmitter adrenaline stimulates your fight-or-flight state of the nervous system in response to stressful or exciting situations. Too much adrenaline can contribute to manic behaviors, paranoia, ADHD, and cardiac arrest. Too little adrenaline leads to low energy and depression.

Essential oils like black pepper, fennel, grapefruit, jasmine, and rose have been shown to modulate adrenaline levels. For example, inhalation of rose essential oil helps calm the excitatory neurotransmitter adrenaline and decreases its levels by 30 percent. In contrast, black pepper essential oil significantly increases adrenaline levels on inhalation.

Noradrenaline (Norepinephrine)

Noradrenaline affects attention and responding actions in your brain. A surplus contributes to anxiety; a deficit can be linked with mental disorders like depression.

Research has found that essential oils possess anxiolytic, or anxiety inhibiting properties that lower levels of noradrenaline to calm anxiety. A study called "Olfactory Influences on Mood and Autonomic, Endocrine, and Immune Function," published in *Psychoneuroendocrinology* in 2008, found clear and consistent evidence that lemon oil inhalation enhances positive mood and increases the release of noradrenaline.

Dopamine

The pleasure-and-reward neurotransmitter dopamine can be both excitatory and inhibitory. It helps you feel energized, happy, alert, and in control. Too much can make you overly competitive, impulsive, or aggressive. Low dopamine correlates with depression, a lack of concentration, poor motivation, and general apathy. Addictive substances like amphetamines, cocaine, and opiates mimic your body's dopamine response.

Modulating essential oils such as lavender, lemon, oregano, rosemary, and thyme administered through inhalation or used topically can help balance your dopamine levels. In a 2013 article, researchers at Xiamen University, China, reported, "Most studies, as well as clinically applied experience, have indicated that various essential oils, such as lavender, lemon and bergamot can help to relieve stress, anxiety, depression and other mood disorders. Most notably, inhalation of essential oils can communicate signals to the olfactory system and stimulate the brain to exert neurotransmitters (e.g. serotonin and dopamine) thereby further regulating mood."

Serotonin

The neurotransmitter serotonin triggers feelings of joy, well-being, and contentment. It regulates mood, sleep, memory, appetite, and social behavior. Adequate levels of serotonin provide emotional and social stability, whereas low levels are associated with various mood disorders like depression, anxiety, eating disorders, PMS, trouble sleeping, and obsessive thinking. The most commonly prescribed antidepressants like Prozac, Zoloft, and Lexapro work by increasing serotonin levels in the brain. Unfortunately, they work for only 40 percent of those who try them.

Lavender and its major constituent linalool bind to the serotonin transporter, which may help keep serotonin in your system longer (preventing reuptake), promoting feelings of happiness, regulating appetite, and supporting learning and memory.

Smell and Depression

The sense of smell is related to depression. In fact, reduced olfactory sensitivity is often associated with clinical depression. According to a 2007 study called "The Effects of Prolonged Rose Odor Inhalation in Two Animal Models of Anxiety" in *Physiology & Behavior*, smelling rose oil for extended periods stimulated an "anti-anxiety effect," which has been described as being similar to "some serotonergic agents" (that is, substances that increase serotonin).

HOW DOPAMINE AND SEROTONIN WORK TOGETHER

Dopamine and serotonin are similarly structured chemicals that help balance each other out. Dopamine triggers feelings of pleasure and reward. When you see something potentially rewarding, dopamine compels you to pursue it. Serotonin, on the other hand, helps you override that immediate impulse.

Inhalation of lemon oil helps reduce anxiety and boosts levels of serotonin and dopamine. Other essential oils that positively impact dopamine and/or serotonin when inhaled include clary sage, cedarwood, eucalyptus globulus, Roman chamomile, and orange.

GABA

The calming neurotransmitter GABA blocks certain brain signals that can lead to anxiety and decreases excitatory and anxious activity in your nervous system. It helps to shift your brain into a lower, calmer gear and improve focus and concentration. GABA calms mental and physical stress, lowers anxiety, and improves mood and sleep. It helps support your immune and endocrine systems, regulate your appetite, improve metabolism, and reduce muscle tension.

Several pharmaceutical drugs including barbiturates, anesthetics, benzodiazepines, antidepressants, and anti-seizure medications target GABA receptors in the brain. Supplemental GABA and pharmaceutical drugs can struggle to cross the blood-brain barrier, impeding the ability of these remedies to modulate your GABA response.

GABA receptors in the brain are responsible for inhibitory signals, like inhibition of symptoms of pain. Eugenol from clove oil is widely used in dentistry for pain relief and inflammation because it interacts with cell receptors that inhibit or activate brain chemical signals.

Linalool, an active ingredient of lavender oil, blocks brain signals that activate your stress response and calm your nervous system. Linalool is a key constituent in essential oils like basil, cilantro, clary sage, and coriander that can help modulate GABA receptors and enhance the inhibitory tone of your nervous system.

ACETYLCHOLINE

The neurotransmitter acetylcholine helps support your heart rate, breathing, digestion, detoxification, brain function, and movement. Your vagus nerve releases acetylcholine to calm pain and inflammation. As the primary chemical messenger between your gut and your brain, it supports the movement of food through the digestive tract. An increase in acetylcholine levels in your brain often correlates with improved cognitive function, including enhanced executive function (planning and decision making), memory, learning, creativity, and motivation. Without healthy acetylcholine levels in your brain, memory, processing speed, and focus become sluggish. Acetylcholine deficits are often correlated with cognitive decline and Alzheimer's disease. New research advocates the use of essential oils like sage and thyme as natural treatments to prevent the breakdown of acetylcholine in the brain. Furthermore, essential oils can "delay development of cognitive decline and improve the quality of life of Alzheimer's disease patients," according to scientific research published in an article in *Neural Regeneration Research* called "Essential Oils and Functional Herbs for Healthy Aging." A blend of clove and lime also supports the vagus nerve to release acetylcholine (see Parasympathetic Blend, page 169).

GLUTAMATE

Known as your memory neurotransmitter, glutamate, or glutamic acid, supports cognitive function, emotions, sensory information, and motor coordination, and it is linked to other neurotransmitter activity. Too much glutamate can damage neurons and neural networks (which could contribute to many neurological diseases), whereas too little glutamate excitation can result in difficulty concentrating or mental exhaustion. Essential oils like lavender can help support the release of the right concentrations of glutamate at the right time.

ENDORPHINS

Your feel-good neurotransmitters, endorphins are opiate chemicals released during exercise or in response to stressful situations or pain, helping to reduce pain and promote a blissful sense of well-being and euphoria. Certain aromas, actions, and foods can lift your mood by influencing the production of endorphins. The scent of vanilla helps to reduce anxiety. Ylang-ylang also stimulates the part of the brain that releases endorphins.

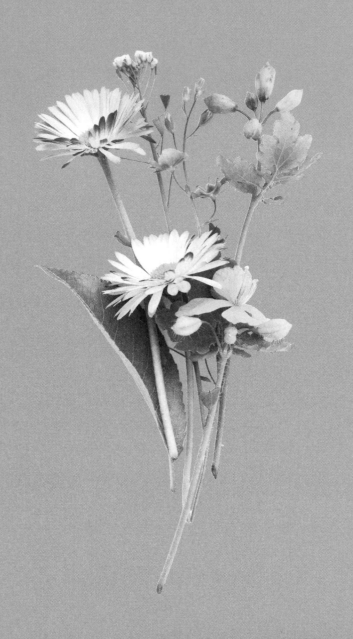

The Endocrine System, Hormones, and Weight Loss

Hormones are chemical messengers that impact how you feel, think, function, and look.

Your endocrine glands secrete hormones into your bloodstream to circulate throughout your body, influencing and coordinating *every* activity between your cells, especially your brain cells. Hormones are responsible for countless functions in your body—from hair growth and skin quality to metabolizing food, maintaining body temperature, causing your heart to beat, preparing your body for sex and reproduction, replenishing energy, maintaining weight—and of course, your mood.

Hormones, directed by your hypothalamus, control your weight, energy balance, and metabolism. Hormones like insulin, leptin, and ghrelin help your hypothalamus regulate food intake and feelings of satiety. Insulin communicates satiety by signaling your hypothalamus to reduce your appetite. A desensitized hypothalamus compromises the satiety signal, leading to weight gain.

Your endocrine glands, including your hypothalamus, pituitary gland, pineal gland, thyroid, adrenal glands, pancreas, thymus, and sex organs, produce hormones that affect individual organs and work collaboratively to control the level of hormones circulating throughout your body.

The Endocrine System

Hormonal health depends upon the healthy function of your endocrine organs. Essential oils can help balance the healthy function of your endocrine glands, boost healthy cell communication, and enhance the detoxification of old hormones to restore healthy hormone production and output.

THE ENDOCRINE SYSTEM

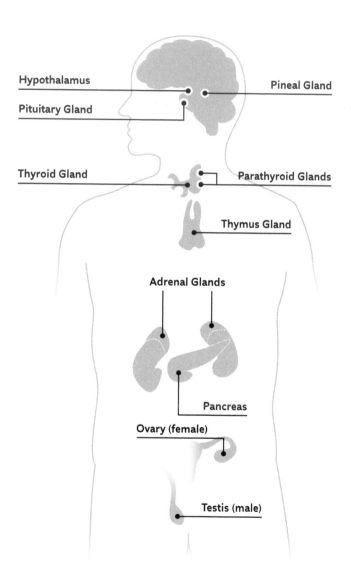

Hypothalamus

Pineal Gland

Pituitary Gland

Thyroid Gland

Parathyroid Glands

Thymus Gland

Adrenal Glands

Pancreas

Ovary (female)

Testis (male)

Hormones have a significant influence over how your body stores fat and when and how your body decides to burn fat for fuel.

If any of your endocrine glands are out of balance or if hormones are not properly eliminated, it can present as symptoms like:

——— Rapid weight gain that won't budge
——— Irregular periods, intense PMS, hot flashes, or other menopausal symptoms
——— Feeling moody, irritable, or weepy
——— Experiencing unstable or unpredictable moods
——— Hair loss at the crown of your head or growth on the chin or odd places
——— Hair feels dry and "crispy"
——— Skin looks crepey and hangs off cheeks or chin
——— Fat accumulating in new places—under arms, muffin top, pectorals, or knees
——— Low libido
——— Dry skin or brittle nails
——— Poor memory or word recall

Balancing the Endocrine System

Your hypothalamus is a pearl-size region of the brain located just above the brain stem that serves as the CEO of your endocrine system. It releases hormones that affect many important processes in the body, including regulating temperature, metabolism, stress response, sleep cycles, sex drive, mood, and energy levels.

The main job of your hypothalamus is to keep you in a healthy state of balance (known as homeostasis). It does this by serving as your brain's internal sensor, functioning like a thermostat to gather information sensed by the brain (surrounding temperature, light exposure, blood levels of hormones, and feelings) and adjusting the resulting signals sent to the body to maintain internal balance.

In essence, your hypothalamus and its hormonal partner, the pituitary gland, tell the other endocrine glands in the system to start or stop the production of hormones throughout your body (through the release of stimulatory or inhibitory hormones).

If the hypothalamus is damaged or cannot adequately send and receive messages, communication is compromised. It's like the game of telephone. You have to hear the word correctly to pass it on correctly. Your hypothalamus needs to receive clear messages from the body, since all outgoing hormonal signals are based on the clarity of these incoming signals.

Symptoms of hypothalamus imbalance include:

—— Body temperature problems and cold intolerance
—— Constipation
—— Depressed mood
—— Excessive thirst and frequent urination
—— Fatigue
—— Hair or skin changes
—— Mental slowing
—— Menstrual cycle changes
—— Weight gain
—— Lowered libido

WHAT CAUSES DAMAGE TO YOUR HYPOTHALAMUS?

Trauma, stress, and toxins can trigger inflammation in your hypothalamus and interrupt healthy function.

Trauma

Traumatic brain injuries can affect the production levels of hormones that originate in your brain. Your brain has the consistency of Jell-O, and any sudden or extreme forward-backward movement or rotation inside your skull can cause the bruising or tearing of blood vessels. Swelling, hemorrhaging, and structural damage to the hypothalamic-pituitary stalk may damage the hypothalamus. Inflammation can also damage the nerves that conduct signals through the hypothalamus, affecting the function of the hormones that help control your weight and metabolism, like leptin and ghrelin.

Your hypothalamus must function at its best to gauge the hormone levels your body needs and send an appropriate hormonal response.

Stress

Your hypothalamus manages the level of stress hormones like cortisol (for more information, see page 108). Chronic stress and the ongoing release of cortisol can exacerbate anxiety, depression, post–traumatic stress disorder (PTSD), and other mood disorders. Chronic stress can generate long-term changes in the brain, even shutting down your ability to calm stress and setting the stage for limbic system imbalances.

Toxins

Certain toxins interfere with your endocrine system and act like hormone mimics. Some trick your body into thinking that they are hormones, while others block natural hormones from doing their job. Still others can increase or decrease the levels of hormones in your blood by affecting how they are made, broken down, or stored in the body. And they can alter your body's sensitivity to hormones. You can be exposed to these toxins through the air you breathe, the foods you eat, the water you drink, or the personal-care products you use.

Hormones

Your hypothalamus produces important brain hormones, many of which act on the pituitary gland, the adrenal glands, thyroid, and sex organs. Others impact kidney function, metabolism, breast milk production, metabolism, bone and muscle mass, and physical development in children.

An imbalance of brain hormones can alter how your body functions. For example, too much anti-diuretic hormone can lead to water retention, while too little can cause dehydration or a drop in blood pressure. Similarly, high levels

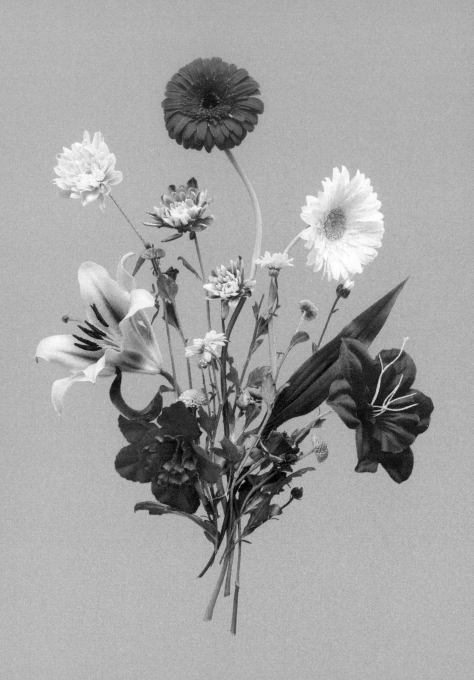

Essential oils can work with your body to help calm hormones that stimulate hunger and activate hormones that stimulate fullness.

of corticotropin-releasing hormone can lead to problems with acne, diabetes, high blood pressure, osteoporosis, infertility, and muscle problems, while low levels can cause weight loss, increased skin pigmentation, gastrointestinal distress, and low blood pressure.

Weight Loss

Your sense of smell can stimulate your hypothalamus to release hormones that help you feel full and support weight loss. Smell travels directly to your hypothalamus through your olfactory system and your amygdala.

Research shows that inhaling essential oils may directly affect your brain's satiety center. Neurologist Dr. Alan R. Hirsch conducted a six-month study with more than three thousand overweight patients. He found that inhaling peppermint essential oil calmed hunger impulses. Participants lost an average of five pounds each month without dieting. Some participants lost as much as eighteen pounds per month.

Hirsch believes you can fool your brain into thinking you've eaten more than you have, so you feel satisfied while eating less. "More than 90 percent of taste is smell," according to Hirsch. "When you smell food, odor molecules enter the nostrils and reach the olfactory center and signal the brain's satiety center, the hypothalamus, that you've had enough to eat by triggering the release of hormones that create the sense of fullness even before you get the 'stop eating' signal from your stomach."

SUPPRESS HUNGER-STIMULATING HORMONES WITH ESSENTIAL OILS

Essential oils can suppress the release of the hunger-stimulating hormones so you eat less. Ghrelin, neuropeptide Y (NPY), and insulin-like peptide 5 are hormones that stimulate hunger and promote appetite. Once full, your stomach signals your hypothalamus to lower ghrelin production; this reduces your desire to eat. Ghrelin production drops to a low point thirty to sixty minutes after eating, then gradually returns to fasting levels three to four hours after a meal. NPY stimulates hunger, particularly for carbohydrates, in response to stress, fasting, or food deprivation that can lead to overeating and abdominal fat gain.

Peppermint essential oil was found to suppress the release of ghrelin. The menthol in peppermint impacts how food smells and tastes, curbing cravings. Inhaling peppermint oil was also found to calm NPY release, especially during times of stress. (See Craving-Buster Blend recipe on page 182.)

ACTIVATE FULLNESS-STIMULATING HORMONES WITH ESSENTIAL OILS

Essential oils can activate satiety hormones. Insulin and amylin are hormones produced in the pancreas that inhibit hunger and food intake. Insulin helps shuttle blood sugar into your cells for energy or storage. As the main fat storage hormone in the body, healthy levels of insulin help inhibit hunger. Cinnamon essential oil and its key constituent cinnamaldehyde make your cells more receptive to insulin and help combat insulin resistance. (See page 90 for more about insulin.) When your pancreas is balanced and can produce healthy levels of insulin and amylin, your body gets the signal to stop eating. Anise seed essential oil is known to stimulate the pancreas. (See pages 184–185 for more about essential oils to balance the pancreas.)

Other satiety hormones that reduce your appetite and make you feel full include leptin, produced by your fat cells; cholecystokinin (CCK), secreted from the gut in response to food; and peptide YY and glucagon-like peptides that are synthesized in and released from your intestines in response to food to promote efficient nutrient assimilation and control appetite.

Leptin signals your hypothalamus that there's enough fat in storage and no more is needed. When leptin signaling is weak, the message to stop eating doesn't get through to your brain. When you lose weight, leptin levels drop. Your brain thinks you are starving, pushing you to eat more. This is one of the reasons it is so hard to maintain weight loss over the long term. Peppermint essential oil supports the release of satiety hormones like leptin.

Cholecystokinin (CCK) helps your body break down and digest fat by stimulating the release of bile from your gallbladder into your intestines. When properly digested, fat helps balance blood sugar and gives you a feeling of fullness. Higher amounts of CCK have been shown to reduce food intake in both lean and obese people. Supporting healthy gallbladder function helps ensure optimal fat digestion and supports the release of leptin and CCK. (See page 179 to learn more about supporting your gallbladder and your liver.)

Peptide YY helps promote efficient nutrient assimilation that both controls appetite and is believed to play a major role in reducing food intake and decreasing your risk of obesity. Glucagon-like peptides help stabilize blood sugar levels to make you feel full and decrease appetite. Weight-loss surgery increases the production of those hormones. The active ingredients of chamomile essential oils have been found to enhance the blood sugar stabilizing function of glucagon-like peptides.

OTHER ENDOCRINE GLANDS

Imbalances in other hormone-releasing glands can trigger weight gain. Essential oils can restore healthy function in endocrine glands. For example, sleep deprivation causes changes to hormones that regulate hunger and appetite. It reduces levels of the hormone leptin, which suppresses appetite and increases the hormone ghrelin, which triggers feelings of hunger. Your pineal gland releases the sleep hormone melatonin. Supporting your pineal gland to naturally release melatonin can improve sleep and weight loss. (See page 58 to learn more about supporting your pineal gland.)

The Thyroid

The thyroid controls how quickly you use energy and gain or lose weight by secreting hormones that boost your metabolism. Thyroid hormones help your body burn fat, even when you're not physically active, providing you with more physical and mental energy. A low-functioning thyroid slows metabolism and contributes to weight gain and a higher body-mass index (BMI).

Your thyroid produces and releases the hormones that control the rate at which cells burn fuel from food to make energy, impacting metabolic processes, weight, energy, memory, cholesterol, muscle strength, heart rate, and the menstrual cycle. (See page 185 for more about essential oils to balance the thyroid.)

The Adrenal Glands

Your adrenal glands produce hormones that support your body's stress response, metabolism, salt and water balance, immune response, and even sex hormones. (See pages 109–111 to learn more about the adrenal glands.) Chronically elevated levels of adrenal hormones, like cortisol, can lead to overeating and weight gain.

Your adrenal medulla, the inner layer of the adrenal gland, produces fight-or-flight hormones of adrenaline (also called epinephrine) and noradrenaline (also called norepinephrine) to help you deal with physical and emotional stress. (See pages 182–183 for more about essential oils to balance your adrenal glands.)

The Pancreas

Your pancreas helps you maintain a healthy body weight by supporting healthy blood sugar levels and salt balance. It helps you digest your food through the release of digestive enzymes and important hormones: insulin, glucagon, gastrin, somatostatin, and vasoactive intestinal peptide. Essential oils like anise seed can be topically applied to support your pancreas to maintain healthy function and hormonal levels. (See pages 184–185 for more about essential oils to balance the pancreas.)

DETOXIFICATION FOR HORMONAL BALANCE

In addition to making healthy new hormones, you need to eliminate old hormones. Your hormone levels and function can be thrown off if used hormones don't leave your body but instead recirculate into your blood. Other substances in your blood, like minerals or endocrine-disrupting toxins, can also throw off your hormonal balance. Supporting your detoxification channels like your liver, gall bladder, kidneys, and gut can help eliminate excess hormones and balance hormone levels.

Your liver is an important fat-burning organ that helps regulate the balance of hormones in your body. It produces cholesterol, which is the precursor necessary for the creation of hormones. The liver also breaks down and removes excess hormones and waste from your body. In the same way a pool filter cleans a pool by catching the dead leaves, dirt, and insects, the liver transforms and eliminates harmful toxins and excess hormones from your body.

If the liver is sluggish or clogged with waste material, excess hormones build up in your system (and around your waistline), leading to hormonal imbalances like estrogen dominance. Once estrogen has done its job in the body, it is sent to the liver so it can be broken down and removed through your gallbladder, kidneys, colon, and urine. If your liver is congested or overwhelmed, it is unable to function optimally and thus cannot remove estrogen at its normal rate. Estrogen can be reabsorbed into the body, contributing to symptoms like fatigue, brain fog, weight gain, irritability, low libido, and depression. Excess estrogen can make your bile from the gallbladder too thick and stagnant to efficiently flow out of the body and detoxify excess hormones.

Excessive hormonal buildup in your body further taxes and overwhelms your liver, contributing to a vicious cycle of hormone imbalance. What's more, if too many excess used hormones float around in your bloodstream, your hypothalamus might fail to signal the pituitary gland to send out fresh hormones.

Your hormones may start to interfere with one another when detoxification systems aren't operating up to snuff. Supporting your liver and gallbladder with essential oils can help to improve their vitality and capacity to support hormonal balance (see page 179).

HOW ESSENTIAL OILS SUPPORT CELL RECEPTORS

Hormones communicate by binding to receptors that are located inside the cell or on its surface, much in the same way a key fits into a lock. Once the hormone locks into its receptor, it transmits a message that causes the target site to take a specific action—like stimulating or inhibiting appetite or energy levels. For example, breast cancer treatments target hormone receptors to change cell growth patterns and prevent cancer cell growth. Toxins known as endocrine-disrupting chemicals (EDCs) can bind to and destabilize these cell receptors, compromising your ability to properly receive or respond to hormonal signals.

Fat-soluble remedies, like the application of essential oils, can be used to maintain membrane permeability. The permeability helps control cellular function and signaling that enhance cell-to-cell communication. Essential oils interact with and help heal cellular membranes and receptor sites, influencing hormonal signaling. Cell membranes are fat loving, as are essential oils. This compatibility allows essential oils to bind to and modulate cell receptors and transporters.

In his book *The Chemistry of Essential Oils*, David Stewart suggests that essential oils not only bind to but also clean cell receptors, noting that constituents of essential oils known as phenylpropanoids "clean the receptor sites on the cells. Without clean receptor sites, cells cannot communicate, and the body malfunctions, resulting in sickness." Phenylpropanoids are found in the essential oils of anise, basil, cassia, cinnamon, clove, oregano, and peppermint.

Unlike EDCs, essential oils do not mimic or enhance your body's own naturally occurring hormones. Instead, they help clean and repair cell receptors so that your body's own hormones, like estrogen and thyroid hormones, can naturally bind to your cell receptors and elicit the desired chemical reaction in your body.

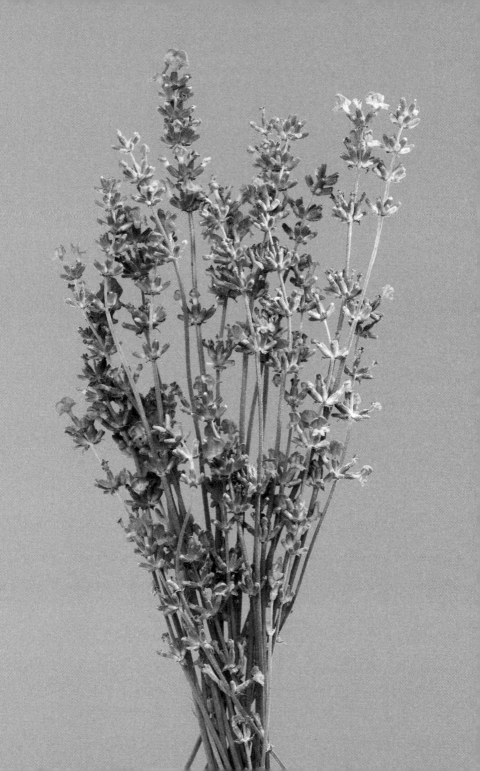

MODULATING YOUR IMMUNE SYSTEM AND CALMING INFLAMMATION

You need to get your immune system working with you, not against you, especially if you are dealing with chronic infections or autoimmunity. Inflammation is an immune response that is meant to be a short-term healing, protective measure.

Restoring proper balance of your immune system and calming brain inflammation is critical to healthy brain function. That said, your immune system has limited resources and can't fight every battle at once. Essential oils can help free up some of those resources. Their antibacterial, antiviral, and antifungal properties can help kill germs and fight off infections.

Reversing Inflammation in the Brain

Do you ever walk into a different room in your home to retrieve something, only to arrive and forget what you were looking for? Perhaps you have had those moments when a word or a name gets lost in your brain. You can describe it in great detail, but you can't recall the actual word. It's as if the word is on the tip of your tongue, but somehow it gets lost in your brain, rendering you unable to actually recall it. Or you might feel yourself growing more fatigued more easily, especially after tasks that require concentration, like reading or driving. These are all early signs of brain inflammation that, if left unchecked, can lead to neurodegenerative diseases like Alzheimer's or Parkinson's.

What Is Inflammation?

Inflammation is your body's natural response to a threat, such as an injury, infection, or even a psychological or emotional stressor. Inflammation signals a series of immune reactions in which white blood cells and pro-inflammatory chemicals, called cytokines, are sent to repair damaged tissue, as well as to protect you from infections or any foreign invaders, such as viruses and bacteria. Without inflammation, wounds would not heal and infections could become deadly. But as your body heals, inflammation gradually subsides.

ACUTE INFLAMMATION
When a tissue is injured, acute inflammation triggers pain and immobility (loss of function) to protect the area and facilitate healing, bringing in immune cells, hormones, and nutrients. Blood vessels dilate and expand, increasing tissue permeability and blood flow (causing symptoms like redness, swelling, and heat) so that white blood cells can more easily flow into the injured area.

CHRONIC INFLAMMATION

Chronic inflammation refers to a prolonged or persistent low-grade inflammatory response that goes on for too long or occurs in places where it is not needed, producing a steady low level of inflammation throughout your body. Chronic inflammation can exist undetected for years without noticeable symptoms, silently damaging the tissues of joints, arteries, and organs and contributing to inflammatory conditions like:

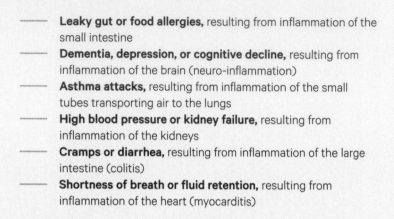

- **Leaky gut or food allergies,** resulting from inflammation of the small intestine
- **Dementia, depression, or cognitive decline,** resulting from inflammation of the brain (neuro-inflammation)
- **Asthma attacks,** resulting from inflammation of the small tubes transporting air to the lungs
- **High blood pressure or kidney failure,** resulting from inflammation of the kidneys
- **Cramps or diarrhea,** resulting from inflammation of the large intestine (colitis)
- **Shortness of breath or fluid retention,** resulting from inflammation of the heart (myocarditis)

Chronic inflammation lies at the root of many cognitive and mood problems, like brain fog, memory issues, low brain voltage, ADD and ADHD, depression, anxiety, and autoimmune disorders.

WHAT ARE THE SYMPTOMS OF BRAIN INFLAMMATION?

Brain inflammation is a protective measure that keeps your brain safe from toxicity and infections. Your brain inflames itself as a way to rebalance, reset, and heal.

Unlike an inflamed body part, your brain may not feel physical pain when it's inflamed. There are literally no sensory receptors for painful stimuli, known as nociceptors, in the brain. Therefore, brain inflammation can go unnoticed for decades—because it does not trigger physical pain. Pain from headaches or migraines is triggered by your vascular system, not by inflammation.

Your brain communicates inflammation in the way it makes you feel. For example, brain inflammation contributes to a loss of motivation, like the inability to get out of bed or maintain energy levels. It can also trigger a loss of function. When your brain is inflamed, it slows down its processing speed, which, in turn, slows down your ability to focus. Other symptoms of brain inflammation range from fatigue to mood disorders, including:

Brain fog. You may experience slow or fuzzy thinking or delayed response time. Inflammation in the brain slows down the firing between brain cells, slowing the overall operation of the brain and contributing to symptoms like poor concentration, difficulty making decisions, and confusion.

Low brain voltage. You may experience limited endurance for focusing or thinking and may tire easily after activities that require focus, such as driving or reading.

Neuro-degeneration. Brain inflammation degenerates brain tissue and increases amyloid beta, the hallmark of Alzheimer's disease.

Fatigue. Chronic inflammation requires your immune system to work overtime, increasing the demand on your cellular energy and depleting you of the fuel you need to feel physically or mentally energized.

Irritability or anger. Brain inflammation can contribute to mood disorders like anger and irritability.

Depression. Inflammatory immune cells called cytokines hamper the release of the "happy" brain chemical serotonin, contributing to symptoms of depression.

Memory issues. Inflammation destroys neural connections that help you remember words and names, leading to poor recall.

Hyper-reaction to fragrances. Brain inflammation causes an over-reaction to stimuli, including scents.

Anxiety. Brain inflammation can make you feel anxious, nervous, or fidgety.

Diminished athletic performance. Your muscle strength is only as strong as the signal from your brain to your nerves that tells your muscles to fire. Inflammation slows your brain's firing speed.

There are key indicators of chronic inflammation that include a range of symptoms.

Pain. While neurons (brain cells) cannot sense pain, pain in your body, like muscle aches and joint pain, can be caused by chronic inflammation. When inflammatory cytokines are elevated in your body, they can attack muscle and joint tissue, resulting in redness, swelling, and pain and contributing to physical symptoms like aches, muscle weakness, or limited movement.

Poor digestion. One of the earliest signs that your brain is not firing well is poor vagus nerve activity that presents as poor digestive function. Your vagus nerve links your brain to your gut, meaning that any inflammation that compromises vagus nerve signaling impedes digestive function, contributing to symptoms like frequent abdominal discomfort after eating, difficulty swallowing supplements or large bites of food, bloating, abdominal pain, gas, constipation, and loose stools.

Skin conditions. Inflammation often caused by a hyper-sensitivity of your immune system can trigger skin conditions like rashes, acne, eczema, hives, and dry skin.

Excessive mucus production. Inflammation triggers mucous membranes to produce thick phlegm in an attempt to protect the lining of your respiratory system, resulting in coughing; sneezing; a stuffy or runny nose; sore throat; needing to clear your throat; canker sores; itchy, watery eyes; chest congestion; shortness of breath; and difficulty breathing.

WHAT CAUSES BRAIN INFLAMMATION?

Chronic inflammation can be caused by an over-reactive or malfunctioning immune system. It may be due to an underlying problem that your body is attempting to fight off. There are several factors that can increase your risk of chronic inflammation.

Traumatic brain injury/concussion. Physical injuries to the brain cause your brain's immune cells to begin the healing process and the removal of dead and damaged neurons, which contribute to brain inflammation. Immune cells in the brain do not turn off, especially if there are already other imbalances in the body. This means inflammation in the brain can continue long after the injury heals.

Toxicity. Environmental toxins such as metals, mold, chemicals, and pesticides contribute to inflammation.

Chronic infections. Bacterial, viral, or fungal infections, such as sinus, lung, and gut infections or gum disease, trigger your brain's immune system to attack, resulting in chronic inflammation.

Leaky gut. If you have an inflamed gut, it will contribute to brain inflammation. Inflammatory messengers, called cytokines, are produced in the gut and travel to and from your brain. To calm systemic inflammation, it is important to calm inflammation in both your gut and your brain.

Chronic stress. Stress releases hormones like cortisol that trigger an increase of pro-inflammatory cytokines in your brain.

Inflammatory diet. Consuming inflammatory foods, like sugar, processed food, or alcohol, turns on inflammation. Similarly, food allergies or food intolerances can contribute to gut—and brain—inflammation.

Hormonal imbalances. Low levels of sex hormones such as estrogen and testosterone or thyroid hormones contribute to brain inflammation.

Blood sugar imbalances. These include low blood sugar (hypoglycemia), insulin resistance (high blood sugar), and diabetes, all of which inflame the brain.

Electromagnetic frequencies (EMFs). Research has shown that EMFs from cell phones, screens, WiFi, and wired homes significantly increase markers for brain inflammation.

INFLAMMATION KILLS BRAIN CELLS

Unlike cells in your body, your brain cells do not reproduce. Respected autoimmune researcher and clinician Dr. Datis Kharrazian, author of the book *Why Isn't My Brain Working?*, notes that brain cells are post-mitotic, which means brain cells never go through mitosis or cell division and do not regenerate.

You have only two tissues in your body that can never go through cell division again, your brain and your heart tissue. Most of the cells in your body die off, and you make new ones. Not so for neurons. You're only born with a certain amount, and that's what you have for the rest of your life, meaning that once they die off, they are gone forever. This is one of the reasons why chronic inflammation, which kills brain cells, leads to brain degeneration.

You need to calm brain inflammation to protect your brain from neurodegeneration—slowing it down as much as possible to preserve your neurons to maintain brain function. There's no way you can maintain brain cell function in a chronic inflammatory state.

HEAL YOUR BLOOD-BRAIN BARRIER

Harmful substances can enter your brain through the blood-brain barrier and trigger ongoing inflammation. That said, healing a breached blood-brain barrier is a critical first step to healing brain inflammation.

Once the blood-brain barrier is breached, there is nothing to prevent harmful molecules from crossing into and further damaging your brain.

These inflammatory molecules trigger a constant immune response, resulting in chronic brain inflammation and accelerated brain degeneration. In fact, Dr. Kharrazian has noted that "the extent of blood-brain barrier permeability determines extent of brain inflammation."

You might think of a breached blood-brain barrier as an open wound, allowing environmental compounds and antigens (molecules capable of causing an immune response) to access and damage your brain.

SYMPTOMS OF BLOOD-BRAIN BARRIER PERMEABILITY

Blood-brain barrier permeability can unleash an inflammatory cascade that can contribute to various brain and mental health problems and symptoms, including:

- Brain fog, hazy thoughts, or poor recall
- Brain fatigue, lethargy, or reduced brain endurance after high-concentration tasks like driving or reading or exposure to certain food proteins or chemicals
- Depression
- Anxiety
- Cognitive decline or noticeable variations in mental speed
- Lack of motivation
- Dizziness
- Tinnitus
- Change in speech, behavior, or personality
- Change in muscle tone or muscle weakness
- Trembling, tremors, or involuntary twitching
- Headaches or migraines
- ADD and ADHD

These symptoms might initially be transient, meaning that they come and go, but as time wears on, they can become more permanent. Once function is lost, it is harder to get it back. As Dr. Kharrazian notes, "If you lose a certain amount of neurons, potentials [for healing] do go away." That said, your best healing strategy is to stop the damage before it gets worse. The first step in stopping the damage is healing your blood-brain barrier.

WHAT COMPROMISES YOUR BLOOD-BRAIN BARRIER?

Anything that triggers inflammation in the brain can compromise the integrity of your blood-brain barrier. Inflammation triggers a chemical cascade that makes your tight junctions—the adhesive seals between your cells—less tight and more permeable. There are many factors that contribute to brain inflammation.

Stress. Stress releases cortisol, which triggers an inflammatory reaction, elevating levels of zonulin, a small protein produced in the gut that regulates your tight junctions, making your blood-brain barrier more permeable.

Trauma. Any direct physical injury to your brain, like a traumatic brain injury or stroke, can physically damage your blood-brain barrier. When brain cells are injured or damaged, they release inflammatory signals, making the blood-brain barrier more permeable, so immune cells can access the brain and clean up debris released by injured brain cells. If this debris is not cleaned up and removed, it will trigger an additional immune response.

Infections. Any kind of viral, bacterial, parasitic, or fungal infection can compromise the integrity of your blood-brain barrier. Research published in the *Medical Science Monitor* details how the "protective effect of the blood-brain barrier is lost during bacterial and viral infections" triggering "an increase in the permeability of the blood-brain barrier and/or direct invasion of the brain by microorganisms." This is one reason meningitis is so dangerous—it disrupts the tight packing of the brain cells, according to researcher Lisa Craig of Simon Fraser University. "This permits the bacteria to slip between the cells and gain access to the space between the brain and its surrounding membranes. There, the bacteria induce an inflammatory response that leads to an accumulation of fluids that puts pressure on the brain."

Mold. Research has found that fungal infections like mold, and its toxic by-products known as mycotoxins, reduce the integrity of the blood-brain barrier.

Toxins. Heavy metals are not supposed to cross the blood-brain barrier, since they are extremely neurotoxic. Environmental exposure to metals through some vaccines, amalgams, and chemtrails (nanoparticles of aluminum) can bypass the blood-brain barrier or be sequestered in and therefore damaging to brain barriers.

Lack of sleep. Sleep is critical for healing your blood-brain barrier. Sleep deficit has been shown to impair the functioning of the blood-brain barrier and increase its permeability. Research also shows that melatonin can stabilize the blood-brain barrier and prevent damage caused by traumatic brain injury.

HEAL YOUR BLOOD-BRAIN BARRIER WITH ESSENTIAL OILS

Gut and Psychology Syndrome author Dr. Natasha Campbell-McBride notes that the blood-brain barrier is made out of the same cells and flora as the gut wall and it renews itself all the time. Essential oils, with their unique chemistry, are ideally suited to repair the tight junctions to restore the integrity of your healthy blood-brain barrier.

Short-chain fatty acids—the secondary metabolites or by-products of digested plant fiber heralded for their ability to heal inflammation—are composed of lipids, which can actually access the cell membrane. Essential oils have the same chemical composition and work in the same way, supporting the normal electrical functioning of your brain and nervous system. For example, essential oils help cell membranes receive calming signals to heal the blood-brain barrier and turn off inflammation.

The use of essential oils, along with dietary changes, helps restore blood-brain barrier integrity by addressing the underlying issues that triggered your blood-brain barrier permeability. Topically applied essential oils can play a huge role in helping to stabilize and block the overactive immune cells to help dampen neuro-inflammation, so your blood-brain barrier can repair and heal. Frankincense oil, in particular, can help reduce inflammation and encourage regeneration of damaged, stressed, or chronically inflamed connective tissues.

Reduce Brain Inflammation

As I discussed above, once inflammation in the brain is turned on, it is difficult to turn off. Essential oils calm inflammation inside the brain by suppressing the release of inflammatory cytokines; this improves brain circulation and helps heal inflammation from inside the brain. Research from the journal *Frontiers in Aging Neuroscience* titled "Neuroprotective and Anti-Aging Potentials of Essential Oils from Aromatic and Medicinal Plants" found that essential oils "possess neuroprotective, anti-aging potentials and are effective in [treating] dementia, epilepsy, anxiety, and other neurological disorders."

Increase Blood Flow to the Brain

Improving the flow of blood and oxygen to the brain helps heal your blood-brain barrier. This is one of the reasons that exercise is so helpful in healing brain inflammation—it helps increase oxygen flow to the brain.

Enhance Sleep

Sleep is critical for healing your blood-brain barrier. It's impossible to resolve inflammation without adequate sleep because a lack of sleep activates your immune system and triggers a chronic inflammatory response.

Fortunately, your blood-brain barrier has the potential to regenerate itself relatively quickly when given the right nutrients from plants and essential oils derived from plants.

HOW ESSENTIAL OILS TURN OFF INFLAMMATION

Once your blood-brain barrier is healed and sealed and you stop the onslaught of ongoing inflammatory triggers, it is important to help turn off inflammation within the brain.

It is believed that brain immune cells do not have an off switch, but plant and lipid-soluble remedies, like omega-3 fatty acids, have proven successful at calming brain inflammation. For that reason, plant oils, like CBD and essential oils, which are both lipid based, have also been successful as an off switch for inflammation. To better understand how this mechanism works, it is important to understand how plants and omega-3 oils turn off inflammation.

Brain Healing Omega-3 Oils

Omega-3 fatty acids, such as eicosapentaenoic acid (EPA) and docosa-hexaenoic acid (DHA), derived from fatty fish like salmon, tuna, and halibut, reduce brain inflammation. Fish do not actually produce omega-3 fatty acids. Rather, they obtain omega-3 fatty acids from plants, specifically the algae and plankton they consume. What's more, your body can make EPA and DHA out of another omega-3 fatty acid called alpha-linolenic acid (ALA), which is found in a number of plants, such as walnuts, flaxseeds, chia seeds, and soybeans. Plant-based diets enhance our ability to efficiently convert ALA to EPA and DHA.

Omega-3 fatty acids, like EPA and DHA, calm brain inflammation by calming the cell membrane's response to inflammation. They are abundant components of brain cell membranes and have powerful anti-inflammatory functions within the body. As such, they help preserve the health of your brain cell membranes and facilitate communication between your brain cells.

Omega-3 fatty acids appear to interfere with intracellular messengers that signal an inflammatory response. When cells are activated by external stimuli, like toxins, stress, viruses, or infections, cell membranes release arachidonic acid to trigger an inflammatory immune response. Omega-3 oils and plant oils, like CBD and essential oils, provide gentle, natural pathways to help neutralize and calm the signaling or communication within and between cells, which, in turn, can calm your inflammatory response.

A 2008 study on the science behind dietary omega-3 fatty acids describes how they can bind to cell receptors and help calm communication between cells (intracellular signaling pathways); this calms the release of inflammatory messengers (cytokines) that amp up inflammation. Several nonsteroidal anti-inflammatory pharmaceutical drugs target the same mechanism to reduce inflammation.

The Vagus Nerve: The Anti-Inflammatory Pathway

Your vagus nerve serves as the detection system and off switch for inflammation. Known as your inflammatory reflex, the vagus nerve connects to your organs and tissues that release inflammatory signals. (See page 23 for more about the vagus nerve.)

These signals, like pro-inflammatory cytokines or a substance called tumor necrosis factor (TNF), released from the immune cells in your spleen, alert your vagus nerve to release the anti-inflammatory neurotransmitter acetylcholine. Acetylcholine acts as a brake on inflammation in your body, inhibiting the production of these pro-inflammatory signals.

This inflammatory reflex is dependent upon healthy vagus nerve signals. When your vagus nerve is less responsive, it operates at a lower capacity, contributing to systemic inflammation. Stimulating your vagus nerve with essential oils makes it more responsive and turns down inflammation in your body and your brain.

Research by New York neurosurgeon Kevin Tracey found that inflammation in body tissues was being directly regulated by the brain, with the vagus nerve serving as the on-off switch—in essence, switching off production of proteins that fuel inflammation. Tracey discovered that vagus nerve stimulation literally blocked inflammation elsewhere in the body, significantly reducing systemic inflammation.

SUPPRESS INFLAMMATION WITH ESSENTIAL OILS

Essential oils possess natural anti-inflammatory properties. They have been shown to suppress inflammatory markers in both animal and human studies.

Peppermint essential oil has natural analgesic, anesthetic, and anti-inflammatory properties that help calm inflammation. Menthol, menthone, and methyl esters in peppermint oil relieve inflammation. Peppermint has been shown to help calm gut inflammation, including reducing spasms in the colon and muscles in the body.

Clove essential oil has anti-inflammatory and anesthetic properties that make it an especially efficient and effective remedy for various types of pain. Clove is high in flavonoids, plant compounds that have been shown to reduce inflammation in the brain. Research on clove essential oil has shown robust anti-inflammatory effects that significantly inhibited the increased production of several pro-inflammatory biomarkers.

Frankincense oil has long been heralded for its anti-inflammatory, immune-boosting, and pain-relieving properties. Research shows frankincense, and its anti-inflammatory constituent alpha-pinene, significantly inhibit inflammation and enhance immune supporting properties. The chemical constituent borneol possesses anesthetic and anti-spasmodic properties. Boswellic acid, another active component of frankincense essential oil, has been highly correlated with anti-inflammatory and pain relieving properties.

Thyme essential oil can suppress inflammation. It can reduce the expression of the inflammatory COX-2 enzyme by nearly 75 percent. COX-2, or Cyclooxygenase, is an enzyme that triggers inflammatory reactions. Pharmaceutical inhibition of COX with nonsteroidal anti-inflammatory drugs like aspirin and ibuprofen provide relief from the symptoms of inflammation and pain.

Thyme essential oil works to reduce inflammation in a manner similar to resveratrol, a flavonoid derived from grapes and red wine and linked with several health benefits. The main constituents of thyme essential oil, thymol and carvacrol, are known for their anti-oxidative, anti-microbial, anti-tussive, expectorant, anti-spasmodic, and anti-bacterial effects. (See page 187 for specific recommendations for treating inflammation.)

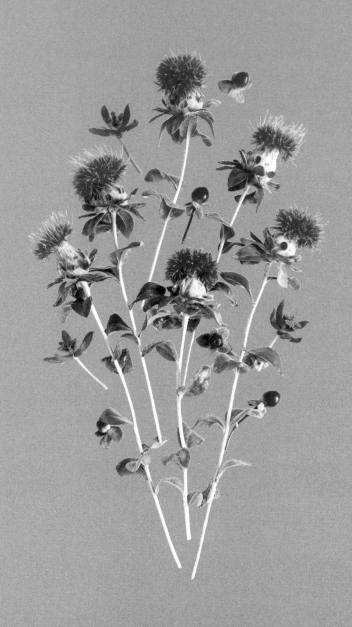

Supporting Healthy Immune Function

Your immune system protects you from harmful substances, known as antigens. These antigens can include foods, chemicals, bacteria, viruses, fungi, parasites, or environmental toxins.

A healthy immune system should prevent antigens from accessing your body through physical barriers, like your skin, lungs, gut, sinuses, and blood-brain barrier. If pathogens slip through the barriers, your immune system should produce white blood cells and other compounds and proteins to attack and destroy these foreign substances. Certain hormones, like cortisol, or steroids or chemotherapy drugs dull your immune response, allowing antigens to flourish unchecked.

The overstimulation of your immune system from chronic infections or food-protein reactions can cause your immune system to overreact, mistaking benign foods or chemicals as threats, resulting in excessive allergic reactions and poor tolerance for different foods or chemicals. Your immune system can also fail to protect your body and may even attack it, mistaking "self" cells for invading pathogens, as is common in autoimmune conditions, like Hashimoto's disease (where cells attack your thyroid) or rheumatoid arthritis (where your joints are attacked).

Immune Modulation

An over-reactive immune system can over-respond to every threat, resulting in symptoms like allergies, asthma, eczema, multiple food sensitivities, or even autoimmune conditions or cancer. A down-regulated or under-reactive immune system can expose the body to increased susceptibility to infections and disease.

You want a strong immune system, but you don't want it in a constant state of stimulation. The goal is to modulate (calm) or balance—not boost or suppress—the system, so it functions as it should.

Over-stimulated immune cells may trigger overactive inflammatory conditions, like inflammatory bowel disease (IBD). Similarly, you don't want to simply suppress an overactive or hyper-responsive immune system. While many remedies can alter your immune system, it can be tricky to know whether it needs a boost or needs to be suppressed. For example, echinacea stimulates your immune system, so you wouldn't want to take it if your system needed to be calmed.

Using natural remedies like essential oils allows the immune system to return to the appropriate balance and function in a coordinated manner. It is important to modulate your immune system in both your body and your brain (see pages 187–193 for essential oils to modulate your immune system).

YOUR BRAIN'S IMMUNE SYSTEM

Your brain has its own separate, structurally distinct immune system called the neuroimmune system. It protects brain cells (neurons) from infection, foreign cells, and disease by maintaining selectively permeable barriers—including the blood-brain barrier and blood–cerebrospinal fluid barrier—and helps calm brain inflammation, heal brain injuries, and repair damaged cells. Brain cells are either glial cells or neurons.

Glial Cells

Making up 90 percent of your brain, glial cells are immune cells that react to foreign invaders, clean up debris and plaque (via the glymphatic system), and dissolve dead neurons. Glial cells support healthy communication between brain cells, boosting memory, cognition, synaptic function, neurotransmitter activity, and other vital brain functions. Healthy glial cell activity is vital not only in managing complex chronic health conditions but also in lowering the risk of Alzheimer's, Parkinson's, and other neuro-degenerative diseases.

Neurons

Neurons make up 10 percent of your brain. They process and transmit information. Neurons are responsible for communication within the brain and for everything we associate with brain activity, including intelligence, emotions, and the ability to automatically breathe, digest, or maintain a heartbeat, through electrical and chemical signals.

NO OFF SWITCH FOR BRAIN INFLAMMATION

When viruses or bacteria invade your body, the body's immune system orchestrates a complex and multifaceted response. For instance, once an antigen (a foreign invader) is successfully dispatched, the immune system's T-suppressor cells call off the attack and send the troops home.

Microglial cells, a type of glial cell located throughout the brain and spinal cord, function as the brain's immune system, but they are unlike the immune system in the rest of the body. If an antigen makes its way into the brain, there is no complex orchestration, but rather an all-out assault by the brain's microglial cells on the invader and, as a consequence, there is inflammation and degeneration of the surrounding brain tissue. What's worse is that there are no immune suppressor cells (T-cells) to call off the attack, and the glial cells, in their unrestrained assault, create brain inflammation and chew up brain tissue in a degenerative cascade.

The overactivation of glial cells can lead to chronic brain inflammation and a decline in cognitive function. Just as an iceberg builds under the water before you see any ice above the waterline, glial cells become overactive when they are "primed," increasing their sensitivity to inflammatory stimuli and making them more susceptible to inflammation that can be activated by trauma, infections, toxins, and stress. This is one reason that it is incredibly dangerous to get two concussions within a short window of time. The first concussion primes your brain immune cells (glial cells). Once primed, the second concussion activates or overactivates them, triggering an inflammatory cascade in the brain that presents as headaches, pain, blurred vision, and fatigue.

Once glial cells have been primed, they're forever changed. This means that you will always have an increased susceptibility to other inflammatory triggers, like alcohol, gluten, or poor sleep, and you will need to carefully manage your lifestyle to minimize inflammation.

Activated Glial Cells

When glial cells become activated, they begin an inflammatory response. As neurons become inflamed, they first lose their nerve conduction or speed. The biggest symptom of this is brain fog. It is the feeling of slowness, disconnection, or an inability to get your thoughts together. Neurons are connecting more slowly.

Eventually, these inflamed neurons can cause atrophy in the brain. Depending upon which area of the brain is involved, different symptoms will occur. Fatigue is a common symptom. You might feel tired and exhausted all the time because your brain doesn't have the endurance required to sustain your energy.

Depression is another common symptom of brain inflammation. This is known as the cytokine model of depression. This type of depression is often unresponsive to anti-depressants.

HOW TO CALM AN OVERACTIVE IMMUNE RESPONSE

Essential oils can be useful tools to address underlying physical imbalances that throw your immune system out of balance. To quote the old Bing Crosby song, "You've got to accentuate the positive, eliminate the negative." In other words, you need to reduce or calm potential triggers for an overactive immune response and boost resilience for organs that help modulate your immune system.

Compromised Physical Barriers

Physical barriers, including the blood-brain barrier, are your first line of defense, keeping pathogens and environmental toxins from entering your brain. When your blood-brain barrier is compromised and permeable, pathogens from your body that should be blocked gain access to your brain. Compromised boundaries open the floodgates to all sorts of pathogens and other large structures, like antibodies that can't normally cross the blood-brain barrier but can only go through a compromised blood-brain barrier. Similarly, if the barrier of your gut lining is leaky or compromised, food proteins can pass into your blood and trigger an overactive immune response.

Low Diversity of Gut Microbiome

Your digestive tract is the home for a large number of bacteria and microbes, collectively known as the gut microbiome with which we have developed a mutually beneficial, symbiotic relationship. These good bugs help balance out the bad bugs, maintaining a rich diversity of gut flora and microbiome to support healthy immune function. Eating a variety of vegetables supports a diverse gut microbiome.

Low Levels of Immune-Supporting SIgA Cells

Secretory Immunoglobulin A (SIgA) is an antibody found in the mucosal lining of your small intestine that acts as a first line of defense in the immune system, trapping and eliminating immune-reactive proteins before the immune system (dendritic cells) attach to them. This keeps the dendritic cells from being constantly bombarded, which, in turn, helps prevent them from becoming overactive. High levels of SIgA prevent immune system hyper-reactivity. Adrenal exhaustion and high viral loads can deplete SIgA cell levels.

Poor Liver Function

When your liver is burdened by toxins or congestion, it doesn't function as it should. Your reactivity to food proteins increases, raising your immune burden. If your liver is inflamed or overwhelmed, proteins will more likely trigger an inflammatory reaction.

Poorly Digested Proteins

The immune cells of your gut (dendritic cells) can overreact to improperly digested food proteins, triggering an overreactive immune response. This is often a root cause of multiple food sensitivities.

Immune Cell Dysfunction

Regulatory T-cells modulate your immune response by deciding whether to cause inflammation or dampen it. When these cells dysfunction, they contribute to immune over-activation. This is the crux of the immune response and the cause of systemic inflammation.

RESTORE IMMUNE TOLERANCE WITH ESSENTIAL OILS

Essential oils possess many antibacterial, antiviral, and antifungal compounds that help kill germs and contribute to their immune-modulating properties. Essential oils can specifically be used to help restore immune tolerance by calming overactive elements of the immune response and optimizing the function of organs that impede or compromise immune function.

For example, hot oils—those that induce a warming sensation like cinnamon, clove, eucalyptus, rosemary, and oregano—can help stimulate your immune system and boost immunity.

In particular, an essential oil blend of clove, cinnamon, eucalyptus, rosemary, and wild orange was found to be effective in modulating the immune system and inflammation in a study published in *Cogent Biology*. The study also found that essential oils "robustly affected signaling pathways related to inflammation, immune function, and cell cycle control."

FORTIFY PHYSICAL BARRIERS WITH ESSENTIAL OILS

Physical barriers, including your lungs, gut, sinuses, and blood-brain barrier are your first line of defense against pathogens like bacteria, viruses, and parasites that can cause infection and environmental toxins like mold. Keeping these protective immune barriers intact helps physically slow or block pathogens from entering your body. You might think of these barriers like the castle walls and moat that physically protect a kingdom from attack. It is much easier to keep the invaders out of your system than it is to fight them once they enter.

Essential oils with antibacterial, antimicrobial, and antiviral properties can be powerful tools for supporting physical boundaries and modulating your immune system. By helping to fortify physical barriers, you improve your immune tolerance and bolster your resilience to environmental toxins.

Blood-Brain Barrier

Your blood-brain barrier protects your brain and nervous system from any viruses, bacteria, or toxins that may contribute to inflammation and damage. (See page 5 for more on the blood-brain barrier.) Once the barrier is breached, toxins trigger immune cells in your brain to turn on inflammation. Essential oils, like frankincense, can be topically applied to help heal, seal, and repair your blood-brain barrier.

Skin Barrier

Your skin is a dynamic organ, composed of several layers of cells that act as a protective sheath, making it physically difficult for bacteria, viruses, or fungi to penetrate the body. For example, the outermost layer of your skin is covered with a layer of dead cells that is too dry for bacteria to grow on. These cells are continuously sloughed off, carrying bacteria and other pathogens with them. Your skin also supports natural microflora that inhibit microbial growth. Additionally, sweat, other skin secretions, and mucous membranes contribute to an inhospitable pH for pathogens. Finally, white blood cells physically remove antigens, preventing them from entering internal passageways.

Skin infections, such as hives, rashes, and eczema, or injuries, such as burns, scratches, bug bites, or wounds, can compromise your skin's protective barrier. Skin infections constitute one of the five most common reasons for people to seek medical intervention and are considered the most frequently encountered of all infections.

Topically applied essential oils can help heal your skin, repairing and maintaining your skin barrier. They can penetrate the skin and effectively treat infections. Essential oils can help increase circulation and the permeability of blood vessels, resulting in accelerated healing. It is postulated that essential oils are able to cleanse your skin from the inside out of harmful pathogens. Here are four of the best essential oils for supporting the integrity of the skin barrier.

Helichrysum has antimicrobial and anti-inflammatory properties that make it a popular choice for healing wounds and preventing infections. Helichrysum is widely used in skin-care preparations, with benefits said to occur at a cellular level, restoring the cell structures and healing from the inside out.

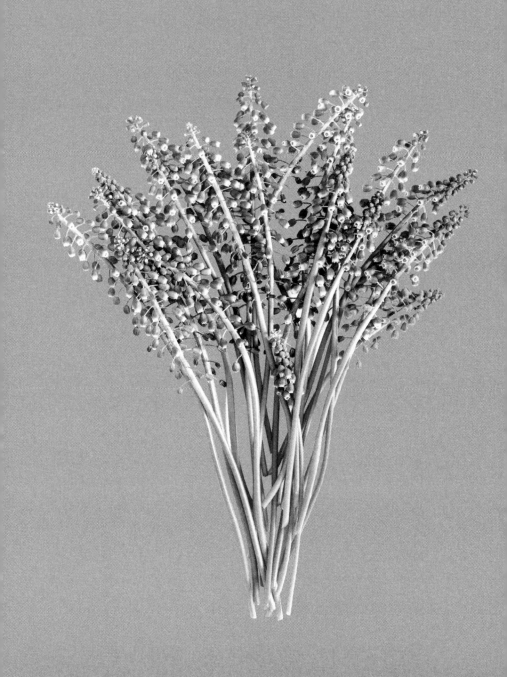

Frankincense is derived from tree resin, a natural substance that is produced by woody plants when they are damaged. The resin protects the plant from further damage by acting as a bandage. Frankincense, and other plant resins like myrrh, support similar functions in the human body. Research has found that frankincense helps repair your skin barrier, heal scars and wounds, and treat dry skin.

Lavender oil has been heralded for its skin benefits. In addition to healing wounds quickly, lavender oil works to kill bacteria, helping to prevent and heal acne breakouts. It unclogs pores and reduces skin inflammation, helping to soothe eczema and dry skin and even calm the pain of sunburns and bug bites.

Tea tree oil can be used to support a variety of skin conditions, including acne blemishes, dryness, and infections. Tea tree oil possesses anti-inflammatory, antimicrobial, and antiseptic properties that make it ideal for calming redness, swelling, and inflammation. Research has also found it to be a powerful tool for treating fungal skin infections.

Lavender Oil for Burns

French chemist René-Maurice Gattefossé applied lavender essential oil to treat a badly burned hand. As legend goes, he burned his hand in his laboratory and treated it with lavender oil, quickly healing his burn with minimal scarring. This started his long fascination with essential oils and inspired him to experiment using them on soldiers in military hospitals during the First World War.

Lung Barrier

Your lungs inhale and exhale an average of sixteen thousand times a day. In your airways, the upper respiratory tract filters small particles. Coughing and sneezing remove larger irritants from the airways and nasal passages and are essential defensive reactions. Helping to fortify your lung barrier can enhance your body's immune function.

Chemical exposure to airborne toxins like cigarette smoke, car exhaust, sprayed pesticides, herbicides, air pollution, and other airborne substances like pollen or mold spores can compromise the integrity of the tight junctions in your lung barrier. Exposure to mold and mold mycotoxins creates a constant assault on your lung barrier, a condition Harvard researcher and clinician Dr. Datis Kharrazian calls "leaky lungs," where mold enters your body through your lungs, then spreads through your lymphatic system.

Symptoms like asthma, frequent coughing, or respiratory issues, like difficulty breathing or frequent clearing of the throat, may indicate compromised function. If lung function is compromised, you might notice you feel worse on days when air quality is compromised. An easy self-assessment is to take two deep breaths, inhaling and exhaling deeply. If these deep breaths trigger a cough reflex, you might consider supporting your lung epithelium by inhaling essential oils that help strengthen the lung barrier, like cypress.

Cypress essential oil has demonstrated protective properties that neutralize threats to the lung lining. Cypress oil calms the respiratory system, clearing congestion, eliminating phlegm, and exhibiting antispasmodic and antibacterial properties that can support severe respiratory conditions like asthma and bronchitis along with respiratory infections caused by bacterial overgrowth.

Essential oils also possess expectorant properties that help expel mucus out of your body and support respiratory detoxification. For example, eucalyptus oil is a potent antiseptic, expectorant, and decongestant that can help clean and strengthen the lungs. Peppermint essential oil possesses expectorant qualities that may help alleviate upper-respiratory congestion caused by asthma, bronchitis, allergies, cold, or flu.

Sinus Barrier

Your sinuses and nasopharynx pathways connect your nose to your mouth. They are lined with mucous membranes to keep pathogens from entering your body. Within your nasal cavity you have tiny, hairlike structures called cilia that line the inside of your sinuses. These cilia move back and forth to push mucus around. This is how mucus gets from these cavities into either the back of the throat or to the nose, where it can be blown out.

When your sinuses are inflamed, thick mucus fills your nasal cavities (where mucus should drain from your nose through the hollow cavities in your skull). Inflamed tissues swell and block drainage openings, including those into the neck, so that fluid can no longer escape. This then leads to symptoms of sinusitis (or inflammation of the sinuses), headaches, facial pressure, and even toothaches from surrounding nerve impingement.

Essentials oils can easily permeate your nasal cavities to loosen mucus and promote drainage. Blue tansy essential oil may help modulate the immune response by reducing excess histamine excretion in your sinuses and calming the inflammation to better support your sinus barrier. (See pages 189–190 for tips on treating nasal congestion.)

What Is Histamine?

Histamine is a chemical compound released by the cells in response to injury and allergic or inflammatory reactions, causing the contraction of smooth muscle and the dilation of capillaries. While the release of histamine is a normal defense mechanism, an exaggerated histamine response can bind to cell-receptor sites, causing irritation and chronic inflammation. This inflammatory response can cause sneezing; runny nose; watery, red, itchy eyes; rashes; and breathing troubles such as wheezing, severe coughs, asthma, or hiccups. Because histamine performs critical functions in the body, you want to balance, not block, the histamine response. Essential oils and other plant-based remedies like quercetin help modulate histamine release (see page 189).

Intestinal Barrier

Eighty percent of your immune system resides in your gut. Your intestinal lining and epithelial cells serve as a physical barrier and the first line of defense, preventing dysbiosis (an imbalance of the gut flora where harmful bacteria outnumber beneficial bacteria) and any toxins, undigested food molecules, parasites, yeast, and other antigens you might swallow from passing into your bloodstream.

A healthy gut maintains a proper balance of bacteria in the intestines, supporting the immune functions in the epithelial cells, and making the gut more acidic and hostile to invading bacteria. Healthy flora also compete with potential pathogens for space and food. If your healthy gut bacteria are already using all the resources available, there's nothing left to feed the bad guys. Healthy gut bacteria also help to modulate the inflammatory immune response and neutralize toxic substances.

Your intestines are lined with a mucosal barrier that plays a key role in optimal immune function. It can be damaged by antibiotics, food intolerances, and other digestive stress. When this lining breaks down, it turns the immune system on and triggers inflammation, increasing your risk for food sensitivities, inflammation, pain, brain degeneration, and autoimmune disease.

Strategies to Boost the Immune System with Essential Oils

Essential oils can specifically be used to help restore immune tolerance by down regulating overactive elements of the immune response and optimizing function of organs that impede or compromise immune function.

BOOST GOOD MICROBES

The diversity of microbes in your gut, known as flora or microbiome, contribute to healthy immune function. Pathogenic bacteria and yeast rely on poor gut health to grow. When gut immunity is weak, yeast and bacteria can flourish.

A plant-based diet with a variety of vegetables helps support healthy gut bacteria and keep pathogenic gut bacteria and yeast in check. Similarly, essential oils derived from plants can improve microbiome diversity. Research shows that essential oils promote the growth of some beneficial bacterial species in the colon. (See pages 188–189 for specific essential oil protocols to help restore the healthy intestinal mucosal lining.)

SUPPORT CALMING IMMUNE CELLS

Secretory immunoglobulin A (SIgA) helps modulate your immune response and prevent immune system hyper-reactivity. SIgA cells are antibodies that dwell in the mucosal lining of your small intestine and act as a first line of defense in preventing an overactive immune response. They surround and contain potentially threatening proteins before other immune cells attach to and escalate the immune response by tagging them for removal. By surrounding problem proteins (or bacteria or viruses) first, SIgA cells prevent the constant bombardment of your immune system that, in turn, helps prevent it from becoming overactive.

When SIgA levels are low, other immune cells become very reactive because they are constantly stimulated to do the work the SIgA cells should be doing. Adrenal exhaustion and high viral loads or chronic infection can deplete SIgA cell levels. SIgA may also be low if you take hydrocortisone or other steroid medications, or if you have a vitamin A deficiency.

Essential oils can help boost SIgA cell levels to dampen immune over-reactivity, particularly thyme essential oil, the main constituents of which include thymol, carvacrol, and flavonoids. The flavonoids in essential oils may benefit anyone who cannot consume a lot of vegetables.

In addition to essential oils, fat-soluble vitamins like vitamins A, D, E, and K and short-chain fatty acids can help support healthy levels of SIgA cells. Similarly, addressing the underlying causes of low SIgA, such as adrenal fatigue and chronic infection, is also helpful.

IMPROVE LIVER FUNCTION

Your liver converts fat-soluble compounds to water-soluble compounds for easier elimination (via urine, feces, or sweat) in a two-phase process. Phase 1 alters the structure of the toxin, making it more immune reactive and pro-inflammatory, so it can more easily be metabolized and eliminated in phase 2.

If your liver is inflamed or overwhelmed and your phase 2 pathway is hindered, your liver immune cells, known as Kupffer cells, can increase immune reactivity to proteins, triggering an exaggerated immune response. Supporting the health and vitality of your liver can eliminate this additional immune burden.

Essential oils have hepatic properties to help stimulate, strengthen, and tone the liver to support healthy detoxification. Compounds in essential oils help keep plants healthy by moving vital fluids and energy. They perform similar functions in your body, helping to move energy and prevent stagnation. When your liver becomes stagnant, it impedes detoxification.

Essential oils are a powerful tool to help shift stagnation and improve the flow of energy and toxins through the liver and the gallbladder. Essential oils can help shift your body into alignment, so toxins do not backlog into your bloodstream but flow out of your body. More specifically, topically applying essential oils to specific points on your skin can activate energy flow directly and quickly, stimulating your liver and gallbladder to help toxins flow out of the body. (See page 179 for essential oils to support your liver).

For example, research in the journal *Biochemical Pharmacology* found that thymoquinone, a constituent of caraway essential oil, can increase the production of glutathione, an antioxidant that plays a key role in helping your body eliminate toxins.

PROMOTE PROTEIN DIGESTION

The immune cells of your gut sample proteins from the foods you eat to determine whether the immune system should react to them. Proteins are large nutrient chains made up of smaller substances called amino acids that need to be broken down by chewing and the release of stomach acid. Low levels of stomach acid makes it hard to break down proteins, which are then perceived by your dendritic cells as an immune threat that can trigger an over-reactive immune response and set the stage for food allergies, food intolerances, a leaky gut, and systemic inflammation.

Healthy levels of stomach acid ensure that proteins are properly digested and do not trigger an immune response. This process begins in your brain. Signals from your brain, sent via your vagus nerve, turn on your digestive function. Your vagus nerve signals your mouth to secrete saliva, which helps break down carbohydrates, your stomach to produce and release hydrochloric acid, and your pancreas to release enzymes to help break down proteins, so they don't flag your immune system.

Your vagus nerve plays a central role in the release of stomach acid. Like muscles, your nerves need constant stimulation to be healthy. Ninety percent of your brain's output travels through your brain stem, where vagus nerve signals originate. A poorly functioning brain does not stimulate your vagus nerve, and stomach acid does not get released. Sufficient stomach acid helps you absorb and assimilate vitamins and minerals from food and supplements. When stomach acid levels are low, proteins are not properly broken down and digested, resulting in symptoms ranging from gas, constipation, and discomfort to chronic infections, parasites, and food allergies.

Topically applied essential oils can help activate your vagus nerve to turn on your digestive function and help your body properly break down and digest proteins. (See page 23 for more about the vagus nerve.) To support optimal brain function and enhance digestion, apply a blend of clove and lime essential oils (see Parasympathetic Blend on page 169).

ENHANCE IMMUNE-CALMING CELLS

Regulatory T-cells (Treg cells) are immune cells that dampen inflammation. Several research studies found that frankincense, and its active anti-inflammatory constituent alpha-pinene, increase Treg activity. Two related studies found that exposure to alpha-pinene increased Treg activity and decreased stress hormone levels, indicating that frankincense has potential immune-modulating properties.

Treg cells also respond favorably to things that boost endorphins, your body's natural opioids. Anything that boosts your mood, or makes you happy, including calming essential oils like lavender, orange, or rose, can help increase natural opioid production and boost regulatory Treg activity. Research published in the journal *Evidence-Based Complementary and Alternative Medicine* explains how essential oils like lavender can lead to endorphin release.

SUPPORT IMMUNE FUNCTION WITH HOT OILS

Why is a cold is called a cold? There is something about colder temperatures that seems to correlate with illness. Conversely, raising your core body temperature seems to help certain types of immune cells to work better. In fact, raising your body temperature by just two degrees can increase immunity by 40 percent. Your body naturally spikes a fever to stimulate immune function to help fight off infection and make your body less habitable to pathogens.

Much of your body's immune response is designed to respond to a heightened body temperature, because heat makes antiviral and antibacterial immune responses more efficient. A fever-range temperature also allows your body to better remember germs it has been exposed to, making it stronger at fighting them off in the future.

Hot essential oils can stimulate infection-fighting white blood cells and antibodies against germs. These essential oils can safely bring the body's internal temperature to 102°F, mimicking some of the major immunity benefits of a fever. Hot oils are not hot in terms of temperature. Rather, they may leave a burning sensation if you apply them to your skin, so you always want to dilute them with a carrier oil (a neutral oil for dilution).

Heat helps to kill viruses; this is one reason why warm remedies like chicken soup or hot tea are given when we are sick. Heating up the body for short periods of time to induce health is called hyperthermia, and it is one of the reasons that healing technologies like infrared saunas, Biomats (pads placed on top of massage tables or home mattresses that emit healing frequencies), and warm Epsom salt baths are effective.

This is a key reason why hot essential oils are so powerful at fighting illness. A popular immune-fighting essential oil formula known as the Thieves Blend (see recipe on page 193) includes a combination of hot essential oils like clove, cinnamon, eucalyptus, and rosemary. The blend got its name from the story of four thieves, who pulled the gold teeth out of dead bodies during the bubonic plague. Despite their close proximity to those dead and dying from a highly infectious disease, these thieves never contracted the plague. When they were apprehended, they were offered a lesser sentence in exchange for explaining how they stayed healthy. They shared a recipe for a combination of antiseptic, antiviral, and antibacterial essential oils they wore in masks over their faces.

In research performed by Weber State University, the Thieves Blend was found to have a 99.96 percent success rate at killing airborne bacteria. This combination of heat-generating essential oils has been found to stimulate the immune, circulation, and respiratory systems and help protect against the flu, colds, bronchitis, and sore throats.

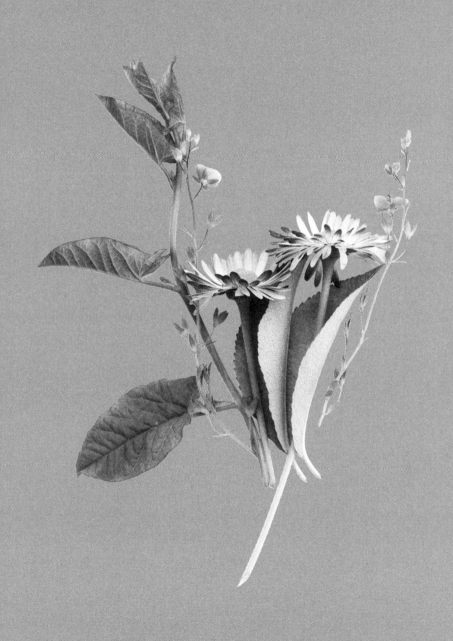

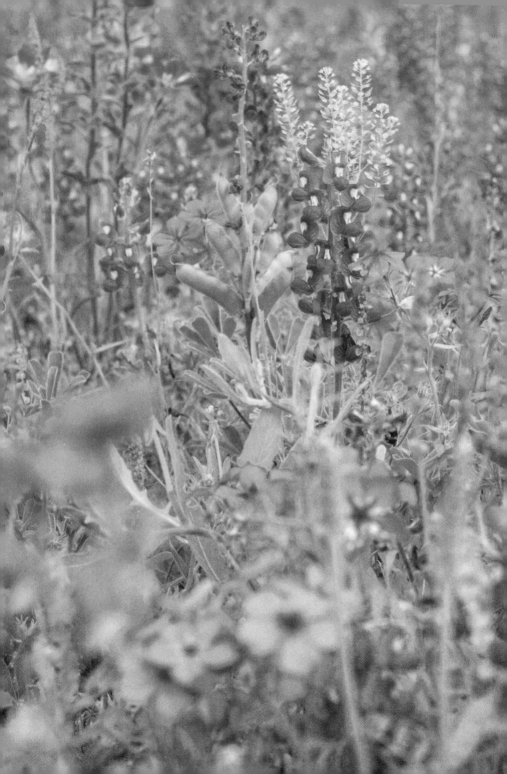

PART TWO

Implementing the 5 Steps

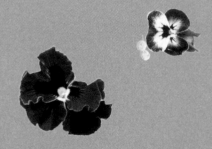

THE 5 KEYS
TO HEALTH

Clients often come to me with a file folder full of test results and different diagnoses after visiting dozens of doctors who were unable pinpoint the root cause of their problems and resolve their conditions. It's no wonder they arrive believing their health issues are complicated and maybe even impossible to heal. Instead of getting distracted with myriad data points, I focus their attention on my five keys to health.

1   Shift into your parasympathetic state.

2   Optimize your sleep.

3   Enhance the flow of fluids, so good things get in and
     bad things flow out.

4   Fuel your energy to heal.

5   Modulate your immune system and calm inflammation,
     so your immune system works with you, not against you.

Balancing these functions can make a huge difference in your ability to heal, removing obstacles that keep you stuck in poor health and allowing your body to perform at its best. For some, addressing these five pillars—and making the necessary diet and lifestyle changes—can resolve their challenges. Others will feel better immediately and have the energy and resilience to tackle further healing.

The first step in my protocol starts with the tasks, actions, and goals that can be most easily achieved. Just as it requires almost no effort to pick

Tips for Diluting and Storing Essential Oils

Diluting essential oils means adding a carrier oil to enhance the combination of oils and allow them to be more easily assimilated into your body. Dilution makes it easier to apply essential oils over a larger area of skin, increasing absorption. It also prevents the essential oil from evaporating as fast as it would if not used with a carrier oil. Some of my favorite carrier oils for diluting include:

Olive oil, ideally clean and pure cold-pressed and extra-virgin, can be used as an easy carrier oil.

Coconut oil is healing in its own right and spreads easily across the skin but can solidify at cold temperatures.

Fractionated coconut oil is my favorite carrier oil. It is ultralight, making it more easily absorbed by the skin. It's also odorless and has a long shelf life.

Sweet almond oil is a good topical source of vitamins A and E and can be highly moisturizing for dry skin.

Jojoba oil is more viscous, with its own anti-inflammatory properties. Jojoba allows essential oils to deeply penetrate into the skin and has a long shelf life.

Avocado oil is rich in nutrients and excellent at penetrating and moisturizing the skin.

Castor oil is not typically considered as a carrier oil as it is extremely thick and known to stain clothing, but it contains powerful anti-inflammatory and lymph moving properties. Castor oil is best used before bed, in combination with liver and gallbladder supportive essential oils.

Essential oils and carrier oils should be stored in glass, not plastic, bottles. Darker glass bottles, such as cobalt blue or amber, help shield the oils from light which help them last longer. Tight fitting lids also help preserve oils for longer.

Keep bottles of essential oils tightly closed and store them in a cool, dry, dark place away from sunlight or heat. If stored properly, most essential oils will maintain their potency for many years.

low-hanging fruit off a tree, topically applying essential oils a few times a day to strategic areas of your body is easy to execute and can yield powerful results.

This protocol also benefits and supports other healing efforts. In other words, it doesn't require you to stop what you are doing and shift gears. It just allows you to layer more healing on top of what you are already doing, which often amplifies the results.

On that note, if you are taking medication, please consult your prescribing physician before making any changes.

1   Shift into Your Parasympathetic State

One of the easiest and most powerful ways to turn on your ability to heal is to activate and detoxify your vagus nerve by topically applying a synergistic blend of clove and lime essential oils where the vagus nerve is most accessible through the skin—behind the earlobe on the mastoid bone. Topical application of this blend also helps detoxify any congestion and inflammation in the nerve that compromises the flow of nutrients into the brain and toxins out of the brain.

—— Parasympathetic Blend

The combination of clove and lime creates a blend that is highly stimulatory and readily accessible through the skin and olfactory channels.

> 10 drops of clove oil
> 25 drops of distilled lime oil*
> Dilute with fractionated coconut oil

Combine the clove and lime oils and dilute to your liking.

*Pressed lime essential oil can be phototoxic, which makes your skin more sensitive to sunlight and sunburns. Distilled lime essential oil is not. The distillation process burns off the phototoxic chemicals.

How to apply: Apply *just a tiny dab* to the vagus nerve (behind the earlobe on the mastoid bone) on one or both ears, depending on how stressed you feel. If this therapeutic dose feels too strong, simply dilute with more coconut oil.

When to apply: Apply three times daily before meals for best results. You can also use as needed when you feel stressed, anxious, or depressed.

APPLYING ESSENTIAL OILS TO THE HEAD

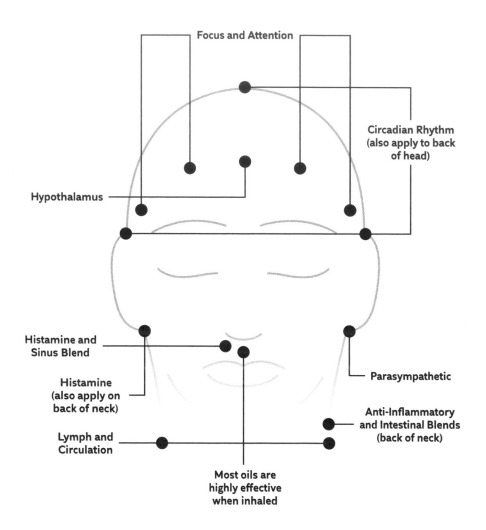

Focus and Attention

Circadian Rhythm
(also apply to back
of head)

Hypothalamus

Histamine and
Sinus Blend

Histamine
(also apply on
back of neck)

Parasympathetic

Anti-Inflammatory
and Intestinal Blends
(back of neck)

Lymph and
Circulation

Most oils are
highly effective
when inhaled

The Parasympathetic Blend can support deeper sleep. However, the blend can be stimulatory and should be used during the daytime to help the body drop into the parasympathetic state by bedtime. Do not apply the oils immediately prior to sleep.

Clove Essential Oil

Clove is a powerful antibacterial, antiviral, and antifungal agent, known both for its ability to assist the body in efforts to remove bacteria and because it is high in antioxidants. It has long been used to heal infections and dull both physical and emotional pain. It slows tooth decalcification, or dental erosion, and corrects yeast imbalances in the mouth, making it a powerful tool for healing vagus nerve toxicity that results from dental toxins.

When applied to your vagus nerve, clove may help increase energy, relieve fatigue, stimulate circulation, support your body's response to feelings of stress, promote optimal digestion, and lower blood pressure associated with stress. A 2015 study published in the journal *Pharmaceutical Biology* demonstrated that eugenol, the chief component of clove essential oil, assists the body in maintaining normal gastrointestinal motility even during times of stress. The authors theorize that eugenol acts on stress-responsive regions of the brain, promoting balanced levels of stress-response hormones that are released throughout the body, which helps keep the gastrointestinal tract functioning properly. Eugenol also is believed to help purify the blood.

Lime Essential Oil

Lime, along with other citrus oils, is known for relieving stress, anxiety, depression, and nervousness. Citrus oils have been clinically proven to normalize neuroendocrine hormone levels and immune function. They were also found, in some cases, to be more effective than antidepressants.

Like clove oil, research has shown that lime essential oil is extremely effective at fighting oral bacteria. In fact, a combination of lime and garlic proved more effective than fluoride at fighting cavities.

When applied to the vagus nerve behind the earlobe, over the mastoid bone, the combination of clove and lime oil can trigger the release of the neurotransmitter acetylcholine to actually slow your heart rate.

Research has also shown that the limonene found in citrus peels and the citrus essential oils derived from those peels stimulate the production of glutathione, an antioxidant known to protect you against inflammation and reduce your chances of developing autoimmunity. Glutathione helps regulate your immune system, buffers your cells from stress and disease, and helps tissues recover from damage.

2   Optimize Your Sleep

If you don't sleep, you cannot heal. I always prioritize sleep in a healing protocol. If your sleep is off, nothing else that you do will be as effective.

Sleep challenges can have a number of different underlying root causes. These can range from low levels of melatonin in the system, which can make it challenging to fall asleep, to blood sugar and hormonal imbalances, or an overload of the detoxification organs, such as the liver and gallbladder, which can contribute to nighttime waking. Once you isolate the cause of your sleep issues, you can apply the appropriate essential oil remedy.

If you struggle to fall asleep or experience racing thoughts or worries while lying in bed, it can indicate that your circadian rhythm might be a little out of balance. Elevated cortisol levels at night turn off melatonin production. Essential oils can help your pineal gland return to its innate intelligence and release more melatonin naturally.

CIRCADIAN RHYTHM BLEND

Rose geranium is especially powerful for stimulating the pineal gland. When combined with **grapefruit**, those effects are amplified. Rose geranium also functions as a sedative and helps to soothe anxiety, relieve stress, and promote sleep. You can also include **melaleuca** (also known as tea tree), **myrtle**, **lavender**, **balsam of Peru**, and **myrrh** in the blend to help restore your pineal gland to healthy function. Lavender, in particular, is known for balancing mood, reducing stress, and supporting sleep. Myrtle and myrrh help balance the nervous system, promoting rest and relaxation.

> **How to apply:** Your pineal gland is located in the exact center of the brain, level with your eyes, which helps the gland register and respond to light to release melatonin. These specific application points help you to best access your pineal gland:
>
> ——— On both sides of your head above the ears
> ——— On the top of your head
> ——— In the middle of the back of your head
>
> **When to apply:** It's ideal to use this blend before bedtime in a low-light atmosphere to allow the pineal gland to respond appropriately.

APPLYING ESSENTIAL OILS TO THE BODY

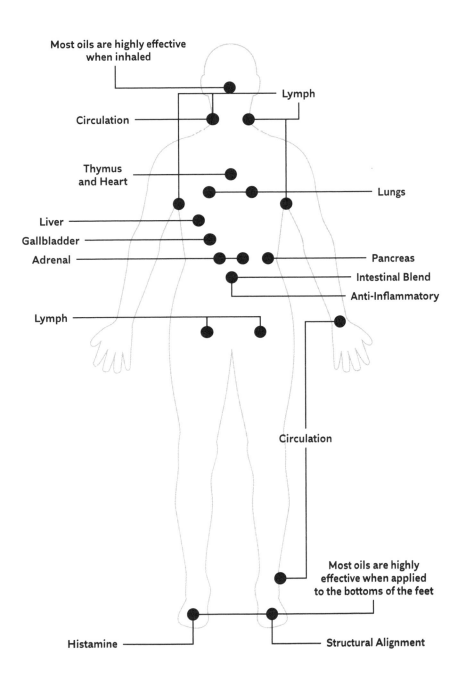

Most oils are highly effective when inhaled

Lymph

Circulation

Thymus and Heart

Lungs

Liver

Gallbladder

Adrenal

Pancreas

Intestinal Blend

Anti-Inflammatory

Lymph

Circulation

Most oils are highly effective when applied to the bottoms of the feet

Histamine

Structural Alignment

SLEEP ISSUES

Nighttime waking, awakening shortly after falling asleep, or waking up throughout the night can often be attributed to:

——— Blood sugar issues
——— Liver and gallbladder overload
——— Hormonal ups and downs

Blood Sugar Issues

Waking up in the middle of the night and feeling so wide awake that you could go clean the kitchen can suggest blood sugar issues. If blood sugar plummets during the night, the adrenal glands release cortisol (or adrenaline if cortisol levels are low) as an emergency response to raise your blood sugar. This cortisol surge wakes you up and makes you feel wide awake.

If you identified with two or more of the symptoms discussed in the section on blood sugar (see pages 87–90), supporting your body with a blood sugar supportive diet and essential oils to support your adrenal glands and pancreas may be helpful. Your pancreas releases insulin to move glucose out of the bloodstream and into the cells. If an emergency surge of blood sugar wakes you up, helping the pancreas carry the sugar into your cells can return blood sugar levels to normal and allow you to return to a restful slumber.

Support your pancreas with **geranium** essential oil or a blend of equal parts **anise seed**, **cucumber**, **geranium**, **rose**, and **rose geranium**.

> **How to apply:** Apply over the pancreas on the left side of the body two-thirds of the way up from the belly button toward the ribs. You can also put a drop on a cotton ball that you place in your pillowcase or leave on your nightstand.
>
> **When to apply:** Apply the oils before meals, before sleeping, or immediately after waking up during the night.

Liver and Gallbladder Overload

During the night, your liver is busy rebuilding the body and cleansing it of accumulated toxins. Your liver is most active between 1:00 and 3:00 a.m., often peaking at 3:00 a.m. When you wake at this time, possibly to use the restroom, but are still groggy enough to fall back to sleep, it is often a signal that the liver or gallbladder is overloaded and could use a little support.

Essential oils like **balsam of Peru**, **German chamomile**, **lavender**, **peppermint**, and **ylang-ylang** support your liver. Combine equal parts of these oils with a drop of **caraway** oil. Dilute with castor oil.

How to apply: Apply directly over the liver (right side of body, under breast).
When to apply: Apply before meals and prior to bedtime to help prevent nighttime waking or immediately after waking up during the night.

To support your gallbladder and healthy bile flow, apply 2 or 3 drops of essential oils like **black cumin**, **Roman chamomile**, or **rosewood** over your gallbladder.

How to apply: Apply directly over the gallbladder (on the right side of your body underneath your ribs). You can apply it under the bra underwire or along and slightly under the right rib cage. If you lean forward, it is easier to apply under the ribs.
When to apply: Apply before meals and prior to bedtime to help prevent nighttime waking or immediately after waking up during the night.

Hormonal Ups and Downs

The hormonal ups and downs of menstruation, pregnancy, and midlife fluctuations can impact your sleep. For example, the hormone progesterone promotes restful sleep. A decline in the hormone estrogen can leave you more vulnerable to stress, making it difficult to calm the mind and body for sleeping. A rush of cortisol can cause hot flashes that alert your mind and wake you up. For nighttime waking from hormonal fluctuations, consider supporting the endocrine system and hypothalamus. To balance your hypothalamus, use a blend of bay rum, frankincense, mandarin, patchouli, and pine essential oils. (For more information about essential oils to support the hypothalamus, see pages 183–184.)

Additionally, excess estrogen can make the bile from the gallbladder too thick and less able to efficiently detoxify excess hormones. Supporting your gallbladder can help return your hormone levels to balance.

3   Enhance the Flow of Fluids

Healthy brain function requires an effective flow of fluids—including the flow of blood, which carries oxygen, glucose, and nutrients into your brain, and your lymph, which carries toxins and cellular debris out of the brain and the body. Congestion in your neck channel and in detoxification organs like your liver, gallbladder, and gut can compromise optimal flow.

IMPROVE LYMPHATIC FLOW

Your lymphatic system cleans toxins, infections, and waste from every cell in your body, including your brain. Congested and stagnant lymphatic fluid sets the stage for disease. Stimulating lymph flow with the following essential oils is one of the easiest and most powerful ways to support your health.

Cypress is a diuretic that helps decongest your lymph and tone your lymphatic vessels.

Frankincense encourages the movement of lymph fluid to reduce swelling or inflammation.

Geranium is a lymphatic stimulant with anti-inflammatory properties.

Grapefruit helps to stimulate lymphatic circulation and the elimination of toxins.

Helichrysum helps to drain congestion and reestablish blood flow to congested areas, making it an ideal oil to support lymph drainage.

Lemon helps to stimulate lymph movement and can be used to stimulate acupuncture points.

Juniper helps to stimulate lymph movement and relieve stagnation.

Palmarosa helps to warm and stimulate your body to cleanse and detoxify your cells.

Peppermint has cooling properties that positively influence lymphatic flow and lymph node drainage.

Spearmint helps to stimulate circulation and enhance lymphatic flow.

Vitex berry helps to balance hormones and supports the healthy function of your organs of detoxification, especially your lymphatic system.

Ylang-Ylang helps to detoxify your body and your cells.

How to apply: Generously apply frankincense or a combination of equal parts spearmint, vitex berry, ylang-ylang, and palmarosa to the following key areas where lymph fluid can get congested to ensure optimal drainage and health:

——— Around the sides of your neck
——— Under your left clavicle (collarbone)
——— Under the armpits
——— Around the bikini line

Approximately 75 percent of lymphatic fluid drains down the left side of your body, so apply essential oils more aggressively on the left side of the neck and the left clavicle.

Castor oil also helps to support lymph flow and can be combined with any of the essential oils mentioned above for topical application over your liver, on the sides of your neck, or on the bottoms of your feet. For example, you can apply castor oil over the liver and on the neck, then add 2 or 3 drops of the blend on top of the castor oil and rub it in.

When to apply: Ideally before exercise or first thing in the morning. Apply two to three times daily.

Note: Essential oils for the lymph work especially well in combination with essential oils used to improve circulation (see below) to help flush out toxins and reduce inflammation of the blood vessels. This further improves blood flow throughout the body.

ENHANCE CIRCULATION

Your circulatory system supports the movement of fluid into and out of the brain. Poor circulation in the brain can affect your ability to focus and concentrate and can also contribute to fatigue, vertigo, dizziness, memory loss, and frequent and unexplained headaches.

Essential oils can improve circulation by relaxing blood vessels and helping your veins contract. This helps more blood to circulate. The topical application of any of the following oils can help stimulate blood flow.

Black pepper helps to warm the body and stimulates circulation, increasing blood flow to your digestive system. This helps to boost nutrient absorption so much that it is often added to supplement formulations to enhance the effectiveness of the supplement.
Cypress helps to improve circulation and contraction of the veins, making it easier to stimulate blood flow. It may also help to reduce triglycerides that can restrict blood flow.
Frankincense contains sesquiterpenes, which enable it to cross the blood-brain barrier to assist in increasing oxygen in your brain.
Ginger root helps warm the skin and blood vessels, improving circulation. It also helps to flush toxins and reduce the inflammation of the blood vessels, improving blood flow throughout the body.
Grapefruit stimulates the liver and gallbladder. It supports the lymphatic system, which helps promote blood flow.
Myrtle balances the nervous system, stimulates the immune system, and helps to calm nervous tension and anxiety that can raise blood pressure.

Nutmeg possesses strong antibacterial properties to help support the healing of respiratory problems and infections.

Peppermint is another stimulatory oil that can help to improve blood flow, stimulate the mind, alleviate pain, and promote energy. Peppermint has been shown to improve performances in cognitive tests, as well as to reduce the mental fatigue associated with performing long bouts of mentally enduring tasks.

Ylang-ylang has been found to be effective in stimulating circulation.

Cypress essential oil is the most effective for circulation. You can also make a blend that is 50 percent cypress oil with any of the other oils. Frankincense and myrtle are also incredibly powerful, enhanced further with the addition of black pepper and ginger.

How to apply: Apply 2 or 3 drops topically to the following points to support energy, brain endurance, and warmth:

—— Over the brain stem (at the base of the skull in back)
—— On the sides of the neck (massaging the neck for a few minutes and emphasizing down-strokes for improved drainage)
—— Over the left clavicle (collar bone)
—— On the wrists or ankles to increase the circulation to your fingers and toes

When to apply: Apply two or three times daily or more often if additional warmth and brain support are needed.

SUPPORT HEALTHY VAGUS NERVE FUNCTION

Your vagus nerve travels down both sides of the neck, parallel to your lymphatic system. Infections in that vicinity can be taken into the nerve, triggering inflammation and swelling of the nerve, which then compresses into your lymph vessels, compromising the flow of fluids in the neck channel. (For more information on the vagus nerve, see page 23.) Topically applying the Parasympathetic Blend (see page 169) on your vagus nerve can help manually override infection, reduce congestion, and open the drainage pathway from your brain.

STRENGTHEN HEALTHY LIVER FUNCTION

Topically applied essential oils can strengthen, stimulate, and regenerate your liver. They can help give your liver the energy and vitality it needs to perform its numerous functions and to keep up with any increased toxic burden.

Essential oils like **helichrysum** and **grapefruit** are good for your liver. I also like a combination of equal parts of **balsam of Peru**, **German chamomile**, **lavender**, **peppermint**, and **ylang-ylang**, with a drop of **caraway**. For example, German chamomile helps to stimulate bile secretions and supports liver detoxification. Peppermint also helps to soothe digestion and support the liver. And caraway can help reduce the accumulation of fluids or toxins, as well as help to reduce lymphatic congestion and glandular swelling.

How to apply: Apply 2 to 3 drops of the oils with 1 tablespoon of carrier oil directly over the liver (the right side beneath the breast).
When to apply: Apply two or three times daily.

Variation: You can also combine the essential oils with castor oil; just add 3 drops of an essential oil like helichrysum to 1 teaspoon of castor oil and rub it over the liver before bedtime. Castor oil is notoriously messy, so you can either:

——— Cover it with a piece of flannel and plastic wrap and apply heat from a hot water bottle (avoid the electricity of heating pads) for 20 to 30 minutes.
——— Wear a ratty T-shirt and let your body heat work its magic.
——— Climb into an Epsom salt bath with the castor oil and essential oils and benefit from layering three healing strategies at the same time.

SUPPORT HEALTHY GALLBLADDER FUNCTION

To support the optimal flow of bile and to allow toxins to flow out of the body, apply 2 or 3 drops of essential oils like **black cumin**, **Roman chamomile**, or **rosewood** over your gallbladder (on the right side of your body underneath your ribs). You can apply it under the bra underwire or along and slightly under the right rib cage. If you lean forward, it is easier to apply under the ribs. Parasympathetic Blend (see page 169) also stimulates bile flow and is antimicrobial and anti-inflammatory.

Cumin and Digestion

Cumin essential oil is traditionally used for digestive health. Research on digestive diseases has found that abdominal pain, bloating, incomplete defecation, fecal urgency, and the presence of mucous discharge in stool were significantly decreased during and after treatment with cumin essential oil. The gallbladder plays a critical role in alleviating constipation. Supporting optimal bile flow with essential oils like cumin can help improve motility and eliminate constipation and irritable bowel syndrome (IBS).

—— Detox Bath

Epsom salt baths help safely disperse essential oils into water and support detoxification through the skin to lessen the burden on the liver, gallbladder, and kidneys.

Epsom salt is a naturally occurring mineral compound of magnesium and sulfate first distilled from seawater in the town of Epsom, England. It helps calm the nervous system and relax muscles. Both magnesium and sulfate are easily absorbed through the skin and into the body's bloodstream. Magnesium is also exceptionally calming and can help reduce stress, relax muscles and nerves, and enhance detoxification.

Similarly, baking soda, or sodium bicarbonate, is an alkaline substance naturally produced in the body that helps balance the body and mobilize toxins.

> 2 cups Epsom salt
> 1 cup baking soda
> 2 or 3 drops of your choice of essential oil,
>   such as lavender or clove oil

Combine the Epsom salt and baking soda in the tub before adding water. Mix the oil into the salt mixture to assure a thorough dispersion in the bath; otherwise, the oil will just float on the water. Make the water as hot as you can tolerate and try to soak for 15 to 25 minutes, two or three times per week.

Binders

When you mobilize environmental toxins like metals, pesticides, and mold or pathogens like bacteria, viruses, or yeast, you need to make sure that the toxins are not only mobilized but also that they actually leave the body. Toxins must travel through your liver and gallbladder and into your small intestine, where they are eliminated in your stool. If the toxins are not bound to anything that can carry them out of the body, most will get reabsorbed in the gut.

Binders are substances like charcoal, clay, or algae that bind to toxins to help move them out of the body. They work by attracting or trapping toxins and transporting them all the way through the digestive tract for elimination.

Because binders can bind to nutrients, ingest them at least an hour before or after meals or when taking any supplements or medications. Taking them before bedtime helps to support detoxification and reduce night waking. Binders can also cause constipation, so make sure to take them along with plenty of water or with super-oxygenated magnesium.

My favorite binders are GI Detox by Bio-Botanical Research and Microbe Formulas's BioActive Carbon BioTox and BioActive Carbon MetChem.

4   Fuel Your Energy to Heal

It takes a lot of energy to heal. Energy fuels the repair of your body's internal functions, building and maintaining cells and tissues and facilitating the chemical reactions that allow us to heal.

If your brain is stuck in a chronic stress pattern and believes survival is at risk, it will channel all available energy and resources that could be used for healing toward survival. This will impact your mood, leading to depression and anxiety, and can also impact your weight. Essential oils can help your brain to shift out of a stress response, freeing up your energy reserves and strength to stimulate healing. Specifically, the energy makers—the adrenals, hypothalamus, pancreas, and thyroid that support hormonal messages to boost energy levels—need to be robust, fueling your body with the critical energy it needs to take on the additional stress of healing.

—— Craving-Buster Blend

This popular appetite-suppressing formula can also be used to calm appetite and cravings between meals, when inhaled or applied to the inside of your cheek. Grapefruit oil and lemon oil help clear the mouth of cravings. Ginger oil is a stimulant to increase energy levels throughout the day. Cinnamon bark oil helps the body to metabolize sugars.

> Coconut oil for diluting
> 25 drops of grapefruit oil
> 20 drops of lemon oil
> 6 drops of peppermint oil
> 5 drops of cinnamon bark oil
> 2 drops each of celery seed oil and ginger oil

How to apply: To curb cravings between meals, smell or apply a drop on the inside of your cheek.
When to apply: Apply between meals to curb cravings.

THE ADRENALS

When you balance and heal the adrenals, they allow cortisol levels to return to balance, so you can supply the body with the energy it needs to heal. This also supports the balance of blood sugar. (See pages 108–111 for more information on the adrenals.)

Essential oils support brain-gland communication by improving the signals between the brain and the adrenals. If you are tired, adaptogenic herbs, or herbs that help your body adapt to stress and restore balance, will increase your energy. If you are anxious and stimulated, essential oils will produce a calming effect.

Stimulatory essential oils, like a combination of equal parts of **galbanum**, **manuka**, **rosemary**, and **thyme** with a drop of **cinnamon**, can help you feel invigorated, revitalized, and energetic. For example, rosemary oil contains cineole, which increases blood flow to the cerebrum in the brain, improving alertness, as demonstrated by a 2012 study published in *Therapeutic Advances in Pharmacology*. Similarly, carvacrols in thyme oil help to lift energy levels.

How to apply: Either inhale or topically apply 1 or 2 drops of essential oils over the adrenal glands on the lower midback, one fist above the twelfth rib on each side.
When to apply: Apply two or three times daily.

THE HYPOTHALAMUS

The hypothalamus harmonizes the activity of the autonomic nervous system comprised of the sympathetic (fight-or-flight) system and the parasympathetic (rest-and-digest) system. Your hypothalamus is located in the center of your brain near the pituitary gland, level with your forehead above the nose between the eyebrows and hairline. It is directly connected to the olfactory nerve via your sense of smell. This is how the things you smell pass directly into the brain. (See page 109 for more information on the hypothalamus.) Scents held below the nose show up instantly in the hypothalamus.

The topical application of 1 drop of essential oil to the forehead right above the third eye (above the nose between the eyebrows and hairline) can help calm and reverse inflammation in the hypothalamus, helping to reset its natural ability to send and receive clear messages to and from the body to help calm your stress response and boost energy levels.

Bay rum oil Due to its stimulating nature, bay rum may help sharpen and invigorate the mind. It helps to improve mental clarity and keep your thoughts energized. It also helps to relieve apathy, listlessness, physical pain, and depression.
Frankincense oil Helps calm inflammation and relieve nervous tension and stress-related conditions. It contains sesquiterpenes, which enable the molecules to cross the blood-brain barrier and deliver healing

oxygen to your hypothalamus and pituitary glands. Frankincense is derived from the dried sap of *Boswellia* trees, grown in Oman, Somalia, and Ethiopia. Oils sourced from Somalia consistently yield a better healing response in this blend.

Red mandarin oil This oil can relieve nervous tension and restlessness, including insomnia of a nervous origin. It helps switch off an overactive mind to promote relaxation.

Patchouli oil Known for its relaxing properties, patchouli helps support and relieve nervous exhaustion.

Pine oil Due to its stimulating nature, pine may help relieve fatigue, nervous exhaustion, and other stress-related conditions.

—— Hypothalamus Blend

The combination of the oils in specific ratios creates a synergistic effect that helps reduce inflammation and matches the resonance of healthy hypothalamus function.

2 drops of bay rum oil
3 drops of frankincense oil
6 drops of red mandarin oil
5 drops of patchouli oil
2 drops of pine oil

How to apply: Apply 1 small drop to the forehead right above the third eye (right above the nose between eyebrows and hairline). This blend is best used in very minute amounts and undiluted.

When to apply: Use three to six times daily to aid with adrenal fatigue or any cortisol issues, thyroid or hormonal balance issues, hunger and appetite control, digestion, or intuition and general issues of safety.

THE PANCREAS

Your pancreas regulates blood sugar and releases key hormones that support your energy levels, digestion, and healthy body weight. Ensuring the vitality of your pancreas with equal parts (5 to 8 drops each) of the following essential oils can stimulate the pancreas and maintain optimal insulin levels. If using for inhalation, do not dilute. If topically applying, combine one teaspoon of carrier oil with 3 drops of the blend. (For more information on the pancreas, see page 132.)

Anise seed can be both stimulating and calming. It helps treat many digestive issues and stimulate the pancreas.

Cucumber's anti-inflammatory properties have a cooling effect that helps balance and normalize digestive problems.

Geranium is linked with "a significant decrease in blood sugar levels," according to a study published in *Lipids in Health and Disease* in 2012. It also helps balance blood sugar by supporting your liver.

Rose helps enhance physical and emotional energy.

Rose geranium is a sedative and an antidepressant and helps soothe anxiety and stress.

How to apply: Apply 2 or 3 drops of this blend to the pancreas on the left side of your body two-thirds of the way up from the belly button toward the ribs. (If you put your hand on your belly button and move over to the left and then up until you feel the ribs, your hand will be over the pancreas.)

When to apply: Before meals or before bedtime to prevent night-time waking. You can also apply immediately after waking up during the night.

THE THYROID

Your thyroid controls your metabolism, including your energy levels. Essential oils like **frankincense** and **myrrh** can be applied over the thyroid—around the neck with specific focus over the Adam's apple—to calm inflammation and balance thyroid hormones.

Supporting the health and resilience of the organs that support healthy thyroid function—your hypothalamus, liver, and adrenals—helps avoid a negative cascade that impacts the thyroid.

Hypothalamus

When the hypothalamus detects low levels of thyroid hormones in the blood, it stimulates the thyroid to secrete thyroid hormones T3 and T4.

Liver

Your liver helps develop and metabolize and regulate thyroid hormones T3 and T4. The liver also detoxifies old thyroid hormones to maintain hormonal balance in the body.

Adrenal glands

Your adrenal glands help regulate your energy production and storage (blood sugar) that triggers the release of stress hormones that signal the liver to break down proteins and fats for energy. This process releases amino acids that are anti-metabolic to the thyroid, decreasing the production of thyroid stimulating hormone. Muscle catabolism also releases a large amount of hormones that suppress thyroid function and inhibit the conversion of T4 to active T3.

—— Focus Blend

Basil has a high linalool content to help sharpen your memory, improve concentration, and promote a sense of focus. The cardamom helps to lift your mood and alleviate mental fatigue, while the rosemary and peppermint are highly stimulating and help to boost your focus and energy levels, both mentally and physically. Research from the University of Cincinnati found that inhaling peppermint oil increases mental accuracy by 28 percent. Similarly, rosemary helps your brain and memory work at top form.

> 6 drops of basil oil
> 2 drops of cardamom oil
> 8 drops each of peppermint and rosemary oils

How to apply: Apply a dab directly over your temples or on the back of your neck.
When to apply: As needed for concentration.

Note: Your olfactory channel travels directly to your frontal lobe, so smelling oils through different nostrils can help to activate and balance different hemispheres of your brain.

5 Modulate Your Immune System and Calm Inflammation

You will heal faster if your immune system works with you, not against you. Correcting an underfunctioning or overfunctioning immune system frees up resources to help calm brain inflammation. The antibacterial, antiviral, and antifungal properties of essential oils can help free up the limited energy and resources of your immune system by killing germs and fighting off bacteria, viruses, fungi, and infections. This can calm inflammation and enhance your immune system's ability to support optimal health.

REDUCE INFLAMMATION

Plant compounds like flavonoids, chemicals found in most fruits and vegetables, have been shown to reduce inflammation in the brain. It follows that concentrated plant essences, like essential oils, can calm brain inflammation. The Anti-Inflammatory Blend may be used to reduce inflammation and encourage regeneration in the inflamed tissue of the blood-brain barrier.

—— Anti-Inflammatory Blend

This blend includes a combination of oils known for their anti-inflammatory and pain-relieving properties. Use this blend neat or diluted to your preference with a carrier oil. Ginger essential oil prevents chronic joint inflammation, helps bring heat, and stimulates circulation, which helps calm inflammation and pain. The limonene present in grapefruit helps to reduce inflammation and regulate the production of inflammatory cytokines.

> 8 drops each of dill and ginger oils
> 10 drops of frankincense oil
> 5 drops each of grapefruit, tarragon, and ylang-ylang oils

How to apply: Gently massage 2 or 3 drops around the back of the scalp and neck to support your blood-brain barrier. You can also apply clockwise around your belly button to support gut healing or over any injured area of your body to reduce inflammation and promote healing.
When to apply: To aid with pain, inflammation, leaky gut, or migraines, apply two or three times daily or as needed for pain.

Dill Reduces Inflammation

Dill is known to significantly reduce inflammation. Medieval knights would place dill seeds on open wounds to speed up healing. Research has confirmed the anti-inflammatory and analgesic effects of dill's key constituents, d-carvone and d-limonene, noting that dill essential oil causes a significant decrease in inflammation and pain. Dill is also a well-known herb used as an anti-spasmodic. It is considered a tonic for organs like your stomach, liver, kidney, and bladder. Dill is also effective in strengthening and calming the brain.

HEAL THE GUT

An inflamed gut can become leaky, whereby harmful substances leak through the gut lining into the bloodstream, causing inflammation throughout the body. To heal this systemic inflammation, you need to start by healing the gut lining. A healthy gut lining fosters a healthy balance of good bacteria and also helps to keep harmful bacteria from overgrowing so your gut can heal and your immune system can return to balance.

Topically applied essential oils, in combination with an anti-inflammatory diet, can help support a healthy intestinal lining, so tight junctions of the gut and the brain can heal and stop the flow of harmful substances that trigger inflammation. The combination of oils in the Intestinal Blend can gently permeate the skin to regenerate and heal the tight junctions in the intestines.

——— Intestinal Blend

This combination of oils supports intestinal health. Birch oil helps to clear the accumulation of toxins and inflammation. With its warming nature, cardamom oil helps to relieve inflammation. Cypress oil supports gut infections, stimulates sluggish intestines, and strengthens capillaries. Frankincense oil is known to repair and support digestive disorders, and nagarmotha oil supports stomach and intestinal issues and reduces pain and inflammation. Use this blend neat or diluted with a carrier oil to your preference.

2 drops each of birch and cardamom oils
6 drops of cypress oil
7 drops of frankincense oil
3 drops of nagarmotha oil

How to apply: Apply 2 or 3 drops in a clockwise circle around the belly button for the gut or to the nape of the neck for the brain.
When to apply: If possible, apply three times daily, 10 minutes prior to meals or two times daily (upon rising and before going to sleep). Ideally used in combination with the Anti-Inflammatory Blend (page 187) for optimal effectiveness.

Note: *Helichrysum italicum* from Corsica is another powerful oil to help decrease inflammation and regenerate the mucosal lining of the small intestine.

THE HISTAMINE RESPONSE

Essential oils like **blue tansy** may help modulate the immune response. The goal is to balance, not block, the histamine response, as histamine performs critical functions in the body (see What Is Histamine?, page 158).

Blue tansy from Morocco is my favorite histamine-balancing oil, but it can be extremely expensive. Its benefits are enhanced when blended with other oils, including **Roman chamomile**, **lavender**, **manuka**, **rosemary**, **peppermint**, **spruce**, **ravensara**, and **vetiver**. This combination of oils can be used to help modulate excess histamine excretion, balancing histamine levels and helping to reset the immune response and reduce allergic reactions and infections in the sinus cavity and tonsils.

How to apply: You can apply 2 or 3 drops of the essential oils mentioned above, diluted in half or more with a carrier oil like coconut oil, to a Q-tip and swab the inside of the nasal passages. For optimal effectiveness, leave the swab in the nasal passage for up to 20 minutes. Try to relax and focus on breathing through the nose.
When to apply: Apply two to six times daily.

THE SINUSES

Essentials oils are ideal for sinus-specific issues, since they can easily travel into the small holes of your sinus cavity to loosen mucus and promote drainage. When your sinuses are inflamed, thick mucus fills your nasal cavity, causing the tissue to swell and block drainage openings, including those leading into the neck and nose, so fluid can no longer discharge. This then leads to the common symptoms of sinusitis (or inflammation of the sinuses): headaches, facial pressure, and even toothaches. The Sinus Blend can be used as a local decongestant to break up mucus, stimulate drainage of the nose and sinuses, and relieve head pressure.

—— Sinus Blend

Use this blend of essential oils, which also have antimicrobial properties, to help resolve infectious organisms such as bacteria, viruses, and fungi in the sinuses and nasal cavity. This blend increases the speed and coordination of the cilia so they can more effectively remove the allergens and other sinus irritants. This technique can significantly reduce the risk of sinus infections or dramatically improve symptoms and shorten the time to recovery.

> 5 drops each of eucalyptus, peppermint, and thyme oils
> 3 drops of lavender oil
> ¼ cup fractionated coconut oil or carrier oil of your choice

Combine the eucalyptus, peppermint, thyme, and lavender oils. Add the coconut oil.

How to apply: Dip a Q-tip in a few drops of oil and gently swab the inside of the nasal passages. For optimal effectiveness, you can leave the swab in the nasal passage for up to 20 minutes. Try to relax and focus on breathing through the nose.

When to apply: Two to four times daily, ideally first thing in the morning and before bed.

THE THYMUS GLAND

The thymus gland supports immunity and needs stimulation as you age. Your thymus is believed to slow down and stop producing immune cells that help protect your body from certain threats, including viruses and infections. Stimulating the thymus by gently tapping on the gland (thymus thumping) or using essential oils can help turn on its immune-supporting properties.

The following oils can be used to help strengthen the thymus gland for optimal immune support against infections, viruses, bacteria, fungi, parasites, tumors, and inflammation.

Black cumin Aids the immune system and upper-respiratory conditions, helping to kill and expel pathogens.

Blue tansy Stimulates the thymus gland so it can help kick your immune system into gear.

Clove bud Stimulates circulation to increase energy and relieve fatigue.

Frankincense Strengthens the immune system by proliferating white blood cells and reducing inflammation.

Ginger Helps to stimulate your immune system, ease respiratory infections, reduce swollen glands, and support drainage of a runny nose or excess mucus.

Holy basil An excellent nerve tonic, holy basil helps enhance the body's natural ability to cope with both physical and emotional stress.

Hyssop Helps support the immune system with antibacterial and antifungal activity against certain strains of pathogenic organisms.

Juniper berry A natural diuretic, juniper berry supports lymphatic drainage, helps the liver and kidneys function properly, treats ulcers, urinary infections, and other bladder problems.

Nutmeg Possesses strong antibacterial properties to help support the healing of respiratory issues and infections.

Oregano The most antiseptic of all essential oils, it helps boost all the systems of the body, particularly the respiratory system.

Ravensara Its anti-infectious properties support the immune system. It aids swollen gland infections and is useful in convalescence. It also creates dramatic results in treating herpes and shingles.

Rosemary Rosemary possesses antiseptic properties combined with immune system and respiratory support. It is a very detoxifying essential oil in that it encourages the cleansing of the excretory ducts and organs that drain the hepatobiliary system (the liver, gallbladder, and bile ducts). This process strengthens natural immunity, stimulates blood flow and circulation, and is used as a general skin tonic.

Combine the twelve oils in equal parts, then dilute with a carrier oil by at least half.

How to apply: Apply 2 or 3 drops of the blend on the thymus—on the breastbone at the third rib—in a clockwise motion for 30 seconds and then stimulate the thymus by gently tapping.

When to apply: Apply morning and evening and throughout the day as needed.

THE LUNGS

Essential oils can be extremely beneficial for the lungs. Oils with expectorant properties help support mucus drainage from your lungs. They can decongest and calm an irritated respiratory tract. In particular, eucalyptus oil possesses potent antibacterial and immune-stimulating properties to help combat infection. *Eucalyptus radiata* can be used on its own or in combination.

>20 drops eucalyptus oil
>5 drops each basil, myrtle, peppermint, and spruce oils
>¼ cup carrier oil such as castor oil, coconut oil, or olive oil

Combine the eucalyptus, basil, myrtle, peppermint, and spruce oils. Add the carrier oil.

How to apply: Apply 1 or 2 drops of this blend topically on your throat and upper chest.
When to apply: To aid with sore throats or breathing, apply two to three times daily or as needed during the day or night.

Lung Support

You can also inhale essential oils to support your lungs, using steam inhalation. Place 2 to 3 cups of boiling water and 5 drops of an essential oil like eucalyptus in a bowl, cover your head with a towel, close your eyes, bring your face close to the bowl, and gently inhale the steam. Or you can apply a hot wet towel compress to the lungs and throat areas.

Essential oils can also be used in combination with nebulizers, a pressurized airstream that allows for quick absorption in your lungs. Nebulizing does not involve heat and does not alter the chemical composition of the oils. Harvard researcher and clinician Dr. Datis Kharrazian recommends nebulizing the essential oils of clove, thyme, and oregano.

Thieves Blend

This blend of essential oils can help raise your body temperature and help the immune system work better. Clove oil, in particular, has been shown to protect the body against infection and can speed recovery from the flu.

> 40 drops of cinnamon leaf oil
> 35 drops of lavender oil
> 25 drops of eucalyptus oil
> 20 drops each of lemon and frankincense oils
> 15 drops of clove oil
> 10 drops of rosemary oil

In a small jar, combine the oils.

How to apply: Liberally apply to the bottoms of your feet and diluted over the throat (combine 1 tablespoon of a carrier oil with 2 to 3 drops of the blend).

When to apply: Apply preventively on the bottoms of the feet before bed. If you are actively fighting a cold or virus, apply multiple times daily.

Implementing the 5 Steps Daily

Upon Rising

Adrenal (see page 182): Over the adrenal glands (back of the body) for energy and **Hypothalamus (see page 184)** on the forehead
Lymph (see page 176) and **Circulation (see pages 177–178)**: Apply over sides of the neck

Before Breakfast

Parasympathetic (see page 169): Apply on the vagus nerve behind the earlobes on the mastoid bone
Liver (see page 179) and **Gallbladder (see page 179)**: Over the liver (the right side of the body under the breast)

Before Lunch

Parasympathetic (see page 169): Apply on the vagus nerve behind the earlobes on the mastoid bone
Anti-Inflammatory (see page 187) and **Intestinal (see page 188)**: Over the gut

Midafternoon

Adrenal (see page 182): Over the adrenal glands (back of the body) for energy and **Hypothalamus (see page 184)** on the forehead
Lymph (see page 176) and **Circulation (see pages 177–178):** Apply over sides of the neck

Before Dinner

Parasympathetic (see page 169): Apply on the vagus nerve behind the earlobes on the mastoid bone
Anti-Inflammatory (see page 187) and **Intestinal Blend (see page 188):** Over the gut

Before Bedtime

Circadian Rhythm (see page 172): Apply on top of the head, above the ears, and back of the head for better sleep
Liver (see page 179) and **Gallbladder (see page 179):** Over the liver (the right side of the body under the breast)
Thieves Blend (see page 193): On the bottoms of the feet

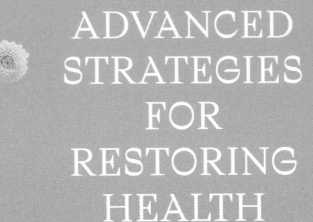

ADVANCED
STRATEGIES
FOR
RESTORING
HEALTH

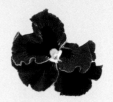

The 5-step regimen can help most people recover and restore their health. If you are struggling with a more challenging condition, such as Lyme disease, autoimmunity, or an advanced neuro-degenerative disease, the following lifestyle choices, environmental adjustments, and supplemental essential oil applications may be helpful.

Decrease Exposure to Environmental Toxins

In addition to supporting your detoxification pathways and your organs of detoxification to ensure healthy function, lifestyle changes can help limit your exposure to toxins like mold, metals, insecticides, pesticides, solvents, and preservatives.

EAT ORGANIC
This limits your exposure to pesticides and herbicides like glyphosate. Adding a variety of plants to your diet also helps support a healthy gut environment.

LIMIT METAL EXPOSURE
Metals, like mercury, aluminum, and lead, are especially problematic because they keep your immune system on high alert and can block signaling pathways in your brain. Part of detoxifying metals includes limiting your exposure to them. For example, aluminum is found in several personal-care products like deodorants, cooking vessels like pots and pans, and even in food products like baking powder. Similarly, if you have metal amalgams in your mouth, you will have constant exposure to those metals, unless you have those metals safely removed by a biological dentist (a dentist who supplements traditional

training with holistic practices to find the root cause of the symptom and support and heal oral health concerns, including safely removing metal amalgams, repairing damaged root canals, and healing pre-cavities).

REDUCE MOLD EXPOSURE
Mold thrives in moist and warm conditions; 47 percent of all buildings have some type of mold or dampness. Not all mold is visible. It can stick to building materials like wood, fabric, carpet, and drywall and reside within your air ducts. Mold toxins can be difficult to remove, both from your home and your body, where it can linger in your sinuses long after the mold exposure has passed.

What's more, one in four people has a harder time clearing mold; this contributes to a constellation of symptoms like sinus congestion, headaches, brain fog, even weight gain. Steering clear of mold and keeping the circulating air supply in your home, office, and car clean by regularly changing air filters or bringing in a more aggressive air filter, like a HEPA filter, can help limit mold exposure and damage. The jury is out as to whether diffusing essential oils helps eliminate mold or feeds the problem. Regularly clearing your nasal passageways with essential oils (see Sinus Blend, page 190) is a more consistently effective strategy for mitigating mold damage.

LIMIT EXPOSURE TO ELECTROMAGNETIC RADIATION
Electromagnetic frequency (EMF) exposure from cell phones, computers, smart meters, 5G networks, and even baby monitors can throw off healthy cell function and undermine your ability to heal. More specifically, the frequency and pulse rate of this radiation disrupts cell signaling and energy production. Children absorb twice as much radiation from these devices as adults do because their brain tissues are more absorbent, their skulls are thinner, and their relative size is smaller.

There are some simple things you can do to limit exposure, especially during the nighttime hours, when you are sleeping. For example, the greater the distance between a cell phone and your head, the less radiation your body absorbs, so always try to keep your cell phone at least 6 feet from your head while you sleep. You can also put your phone on airplane mode and unplug your Wi-Fi router at night to limit radiation exposure. Similarly, pulling your bed 5 inches away from the wall helps limit exposure to electrical currents running through your walls. Essential oils like rose and lavender can help balance your body and offset the damage of radiation.

DECREASE YOUR MICROBIAL BURDEN

Once you have safely opened your detoxification and drainage pathways, it is safe to start killing the parasites, viruses, bacteria, yeast, fungi, and infections that contribute to brain dysfunction.

While essential oils possess multiple antiviral and antibacterial qualities, I am cautious about ingesting any of them to eradicate pathogens. Remember they are highly concentrated and can kill the good bugs along with the bad. If you are interested in ingesting essential oils for this purpose, please work with a trained practitioner so you don't do any harm. Some herbs, supplements, and pharmaceutical medications are also beneficial for eradicating pathogens. Killing pathogens is not a one size, or one oil, fits all protocol. I strongly encourage you to work with a medical practitioner to customize this protocol to your individual gut challenges.

Vagus nerve stimulation and immune modulation both help to support your gut microbiome. Applying oils on strategic acupuncture points can be more effective than ingesting oils, especially as pathogens live in your nerves and organs as well as in your gut. The "spleen 6 point," which is inside of the leg, just above the highest peak of your ankle (four finger widths up from, as you apply the oil; it helps to apply pressure on the tibia bone), is a powerful application point that supports your immune, digestive, and detoxification channels.

Biofilms

While I am hesitant to advocate the internal consumption of essential oils, there is much evidence of their healing potential for antibiotic-resistant biofilms.

Biofilms are protective shields that pathogens like bacteria, fungi, and parasites create to hide themselves from your immune system. Biofilms adhere to and colonize warm and moist surfaces in your body—like your mouth, gut, nasal passageways, lungs, ear canals, vaginal mucous membrane, or chronic wounds and ulcers—since these surfaces offer an ideal breeding ground for bacteria. They create a protective physical barrier of a gluelike film that literally cloaks these bad bugs in an antibiotic treatment.

Biofilm-producing microorganisms are suspected in playing a role in most antibacterial-resistant infections, including strep throat, Lyme disease, lupus, and sinusitis, and are now estimated to be involved with 80 percent of all digestive dysfunction, including Crohn's disease and ulcerative colitis.

Research shows that essential oils, with their antimicrobial, antifungal, antiviral, antiparasitic, and antibacterial qualities have proven highly effective at eradicating bacteria within biofilms, even when antibiotic resistance was in place. More specifically, to effectively treat the microbes that are hiding beneath biofilms, remedies need to break through the biofilm, destroy the pathogens within the biofilm, and detoxify the biotoxin waste products. Certain essential oils are able to do exactly this—penetrate and break down the cell walls of the biofilms and effectively degrade biofilms and kill bacteria.

Plaque on teeth is an example of a biofilm, and the success of essential oil mouthwashes such as Listerine, which contains four essential oil constituents, thymol, menthol, 1,8-cineole, and methyl salicylate, when compared to others is partly due to their ability to break down and inhibit plaque formation.

Clove oil exhibits impressive inhibitory effect on biofilm formation, along with anti-adhesion and biofilm disruption activities. Out of eighty-three essential oils tested in the study "Essential Oils and Eugenols Inhibit Biofilm Formation and the Virulence of *Escherichia coli*," clove oil and its chemical compound eugenol were the most effective biofilm inhibitors.

Oregano oil, which contains carvacrol, significantly inhibits biofilm formation without inhibiting immune function. Carvacrol has been shown to inhibit antibiotic-resistant bacteria, viruses, parasites, and fungi and may help reduce the strength and mobility of biofilm-related substances, helping to prevent the spread of biofilms.

Thyme oil, with its an active component thymol, provides exceptional protection against bacteria associated with biofilms. Thymol is believed to disrupt biofilm formation and reduce infection intensity by limiting chemical communication between specific microorganisms in a large collection of biofilms.

Other Nutritional Support

Nutrients, like vitamins and minerals, are the building blocks your cells need for healing. Nutrient deficiencies or a surplus of toxins can interfere with your ability to heal. The following strategies can help amplify your health.

BINDERS

As previously recommended, if you are mobilizing toxins, you always want to take binders—substances like clay or charcoal that help bind to toxins and ensure that those toxins leave your body. (See page 181 for recommended brands.)

HYDRATION

Water is the most important nutrient in the body. It comprises 75 percent of your brain. Every function of the body is determined by the efficient flow of water to help transport nutrients to your body and waste out of your system. We need to be constantly replenishing ourselves. Our bodies lose 10 to 12 cups of water daily through breathing, digestion, elimination, and perspiration. The body can produce only 8 percent of its daily water needs itself. The remaining 92 percent must be obtained through the foods we eat and the beverages we drink. It is essential that we consume enough water each day. It takes only a small deficiency of water to throw the body into dehydration mode. When dehydrated, the body must ration its use of water. Diuretic beverages like coffee, caffeinated teas, fruit juices, sodas, and alcohol rob your body's hydration stores and can contribute to dehydration.

Mental Support

When you strengthen the prefrontal cortex, you enhance your brain's mental energy and with it your processing speed. The following essential oils can help enhance concentration and alertness, support clear thinking, and help you stay focused on the task at hand, especially when applied over the forehead to the prefrontal lobe.

Focus Blend (page 186) includes oils that help keep your mind thinking clearly and directed to the task at hand. The combination of the indicated oils in specific ratios creates a synergistic effect, boosting their effectiveness.

ESSENTIAL OILS FOR ADD AND ADHD

The following blend of essential oils has been shown to improve ADD and ADHD symptoms:

> 3 drops of cedarwood
> 3 drops of frankincense
> 3 drops of lavender
> 3 drops of vetiver

Cedarwood. Helps to strengthen the nervous system and keep focus in the face of ADD and ADHD issues.

Frankincense. Helps fortify the mind, eliminate indecision, and boost your mood. Also reduces inflammation, which can help lower cortisol levels and calm your mood.

Lavender. Balances mood, reduces stress and tension, calms the mind, and enhances the other oils in this blend for optimal effectiveness.
Vetiver. In a 2001 study by Dr. Terry Friedmann, vetiver doubled the successful performance in children with ADD and ADHD. It is one of the best oils for grounding, calming the mind, and focusing on specific tasks.

How to apply: For best results, apply 1 or 2 drops on the back of the neck, where the brain stem is, or a small diluted amount on the temples, across the forehead, and on the bottoms of the feet.
When to apply: To aid with mental attention, apply two or three times daily or as needed during moments of inattention and distraction. Put a few drops on a tissue and have it close, where you can smell it, when you start to feel out of control or unfocused.

Emotional Support

Essential oils can be used to help shift emotions. Remember that your sense of smell links directly to the limbic lobe of your brain, which stores and releases emotional trauma. This direct route to your limbic system allows smell to mobilize long-forgotten memories and emotions.

You can use essential oils, in combination with breath, to help release and repair emotional blocks, diminishing the pattern of the negative emotions and thoughts and replacing them with more positive options. Adding other modalities, like tapping on reflex points to release emotional or energetic blockages, also known as Emotional Freedom Techniques, and positive affirmations, can be helpful too.

Here is my strategy for releasing negative emotions. First, focus on the negative emotions or repetitive thought patterns that you would like to release. You can do this by speaking your concern out loud to yourself in front of a mirror or to a trusted friend. If you can, try to dig deep into your emotional memory and recall where you might have first experienced this emotion or thought pattern—perhaps somewhere in early childhood. Validate yourself, this experience, and any emotions you might be feeling, including anger, fear, grief, shame, or guilt. You are entitled to those feelings, but those feelings are no longer serving you. So, it is time to release them.

In this process, the exhale releases the hurts of the past. Therefore, the deeper you breathe while smelling the oil and the more forceful the out breath, the sooner the emotion is released. This is my favorite technique: Take a deep breath, slowly inhale the oil, and then exhale; repeat this for between three and seven breaths. You will know that the oil is working when you stop smelling it.

Deeply inhale the smell of the oil while you concentrate on the past hurt or emotion. Acknowledge those intense emotions, and then as you exhale, allow them to flow out of you. If tears flow as well, just allow them, since tears help release old hormones from the body.

Once you feel that you have released the emotion to the best of your ability, you can then fill the negative space with a positive affirmation. Louise Hay offers affirmation suggestions in *You Can Heal Your Life,* but you are encouraged to replace them with anything that calls to your heart.

The process of instilling a positive affirmation is the same: inhale the oil for three to seven breaths and concentrate on the positive affirmation as if you were breathing it into your system. Hold the breath and let the positive affirmation settle into your body. You might physically feel your system relax and return to balance. When you are ready, exhale slowly.

You can repeat this breathing exercise as often as you need it, knowing that the intensity of the emotional memory will fade the more you release it with the oil and your breath. Do note that since we are all bio-individual, experiences may vary from person to person.

The following essential oils are some of my favorites to release past hurts.

Blue tansy oil, a cobalt blue oil derived from a flowering plant in Morocco, is my favorite for helping to release negative emotions and anything that is keeping you stuck. It helps to alleviate feelings of being overwhelmed and exhaustion so you can move forward. Inhaled or massaged over your heart, your throat, or behind your ears, blue tansy allows you to release anger and suppress negative memories that are often stored at very deep cellular levels.

Frankincense, a grounding and centering oil derived from resin, can help improve your body's ability to protect and heal. It is helpful for releasing anger, overcoming grief, and dispelling fear and can be useful for relieving feelings of grief or emotional trauma. To use, inhale or massage over your heart, at the base of your skull, or on the bottoms of your feet.

Rose oil is extremely uplifting and one of the best choices for improving mental well-being and providing emotional relief due to anxiety, grief, worry, trauma, and anger. Research has confirmed how rose oil relieves stress and increases feelings of calm and relaxation. To use, inhale or massage over your heart, on your wrists, or behind your ears.

Even when the emotions are released slowly and gradually, it can be overwhelming. I equate the experience to cleaning out a storage place in your house. It often gets messier before it gets cleaner. You have to pull everything out of your neatly tucked away hiding spaces, look at it, and decide what needs to be tossed, kept, or further processed. The same is true for emotions.

Chiropractic Work

Essential oil blends, like the Structural Alignment Blend, can be topically applied after structural alignment sessions to help hold and maintain the correction.

—— Structural Alignment Blend

This blend has been called "chiropractor in a bottle," because it helps you to maintain alignment and balance within your body after a chiropractic correction. The blue tansy helps to strengthen self-control, dispel negativity, and overcome anger issues. The frankincense not only helps to overcome negativity but also to dispel feelings of unworthiness. The rosewood helps you feel safe and face your fears, while the spruce helps eliminate emotional blocks and reduce mental fatigue.

> 6 drops of blue tansy oil
> 7 drops of frankincense oil
> 2 drops of rosewood oil
> 15 drops of spruce oil

How to apply: Apply 2 to 3 drops over the liver (right side of the body under the breast). You can also apply with a castor oil pack over the liver or place a drop or two on the palms, rub hands together, cover your nose, and inhale.

When to apply: To aid with the release of anger, irritation, and frustration, apply two to three times daily or as needed during grumpy moments. Put a few drops on a tissue and have it close, where you can smell it, when you start to feel out of control.

Next Steps

I hope the five steps outlined in part two have helped you shift your body into balance, allowing you to easily eliminate toxins, calm inflammation, restore sleep, enhance energy, boost immunity, and start feeling like your best self again. I know this has been the case for myself and many of my clients. When we help the body return to balance, we can quickly regain our brain power, regain our energy, and begin to reclaim our health.

Congratulations on taking these first steps. I would love to continue to support you in the next steps of your healing journey with additional information and resources. You can find downloadable checklists, book updates, and ongoing support at www.boostthebrainbook.com/resources.

I hope to see you there!

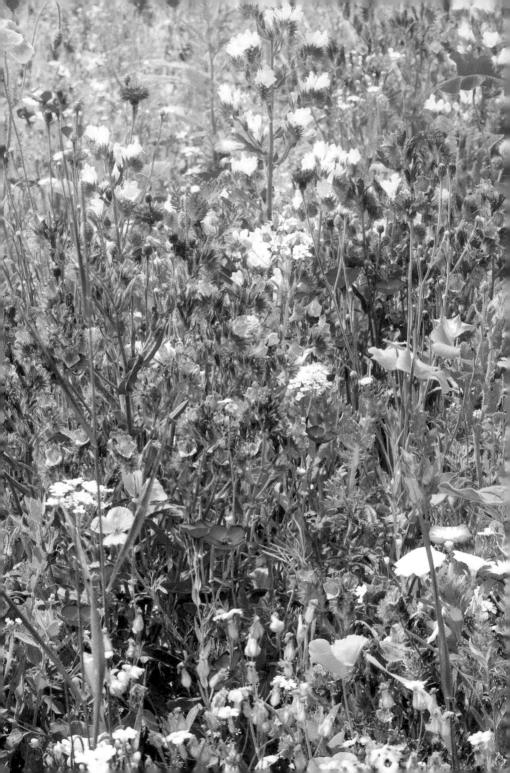

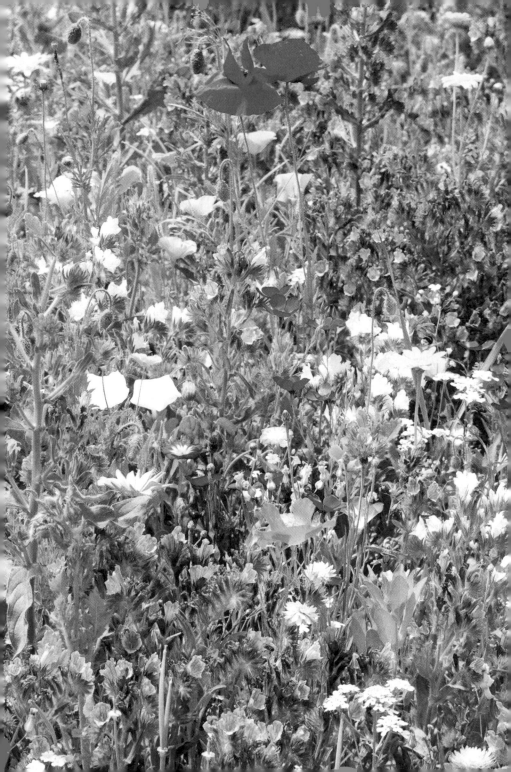

AUTHOR'S NOTE

Thank you for joining me on the journey to boost the brain and heal the body with essential oils. For many of you, the strategies in this book will help regenerate brain health and restore your energy, mood, and focus. For others, it may be a starting point that you can build upon to begin to unravel chronic health challenges or explore greater healing potentials with essential oils. There are many paths to healing, and I hope this book has helped empower you with more natural, non-invasive tools, like essential oils.

I'm deeply honored to be a participant in your journey to health and I hope we can stay connected. My passion for using essential oils to heal the brain and boost the body grows deeper with every new discovery, every success story, and every client challenge that leads me to discover more solutions.

I would love to connect with you to learn about your successes and challenges and also share new research and healing strategies. Please stay in touch. You can find me on social media and by visiting my website.

In vibrant health,
Jodi Cohen
www.vibrantblueoils.com
www.boostthebrainbook.com/resources
https://www.facebook.com/vibrantblueoils/
https://www.facebook.com/groups/VibrantBlueOilsDiscussionGroup/
@vibrantblueoils

ACKNOWLEDGMENTS

I want to acknowledge and thank you, dear reader, for opening your mind and your heart to the content in this book. It was truly a work of love.

The knowledge and information shared in this book was gleaned from my own healing journey after the tragic loss of my twelve-year-old son, Max. He inspired me to learn and grow throughout his short life, and that legacy continues past his untimely death. While I would never wish the pain and intensity of my experience on anyone, I do hope that the 5 keys to health I discovered on this journey will lessen the mental, physical, and emotional pain you may be facing in your own life.

Thank you to my beautiful and amazing daughter, Carly Cohen; my mother, Barbara Sternoff; my sister Lisa Feldman; and my emotional support team: Liz Hletko, Naomi Panzer, Sarah Gomez, Dr. Christine Schaffner, and the late Nicole Condit Duncan, for your unconditional love, insight, patience, loyalty, and support throughout this journey and this lifetime. Friendship is the best medicine and your intelligence, compassion, humor, and insight have carried me through many dark hours.

This book would not have been possible without the guidance and support of Kim Keller, Julie Bennett, and Isabelle Gioffredi at Ten Speed Press and Celeste Fine, and Jaidree Braddix at Park & Fine. Thank you also to Courtney Kenney, Odette Fleming, Jana Branson, and the entire Random House marketing team for your wonderful ideas and ongoing support, and Lisi and Rob Wolf for your beautiful photographs!

Thank you to my amazing team at Vibrant Blue Oils, including Darcie Purcell, Tressa Beheim, Rebecca Odle, Jill Hutchins, Anna Moren, Heather Larson, Kate Mackie, Christy Olsen, Jen Ward, Charissa Wilson, and Dmitriy Agadzhanov. You are the wind beneath my wings, and it is an honor and a privilege to work with you every day.

I am also immensely grateful for the brilliance and kindness of my professional confidents and cheerleaders, including Mary Agnes Antonopoulos, Peter Hoppenfeld, Evan Hirsch, Heidi Hanna, Cassie Bjork, Amy Stark, Debi Silber, Elisa Song, Julie Matthews, Terry Wahls, Deanna Minich, Michelle Norris, Keesha Ewers, Wendy Myers, Randall Zamcheck, Brett Fairall, Katie Packwood, Anne Fischer Silva, Margaret Floyd Barry, Donna Mosher, Bridgit Danner, Todd Watts, Lloyd Burrell, Josh Shideler, Miriam Mosley, Maya Shetreat, Niki Gratix, Anna Cabeca, Robyn Openshaw, and JJ Virgin.

Thank you to Andrea Dahlman, Renee Herst, Amy Lewis, Amy Friedman, Jen Rice, Caroline Gangi, Carolyn Lese, Margaret Castellanos, Erica Keswin, Josh Orenstein, Alison Tintle, Cassandra Western, Gini Powers, Suzi LeVine,

Wendy Carlyle, Lynn Resnick, Lisa Loop, Matt Haba, Nick Jenkins, Lauren Vogt, and Karen Andonian for your friendship and support. To my college friends, Laurie Siebert, Susan Feddersen, Susie Flynn, Kristi Roemer, Sue Naegle, Whitney Vicca: thank for reminding me to have fun. To my bonus family, Ruby, Carolyn, Leah, and Talia Namdar-Cohen; Dan, Mara, Sam, Ethan, and Sasha Cohen; Helen Cohen and Anna Schwartz-Cohen; Gail, Jonathon, Emanuel, Michal, Gedalia, Nava, and Jacob Schorsch; Lisa, Tom, Michaela, Hana, and Avi Cohen-Fuentes; Peter and Nancy Caigan; and Boris Feldman: thank you for keeping Max alive in your hearts. To Max's surviving friends and their families, especially Julian and Grace Paulus; Paul and Octavio Rosales; Joyce Aoyama; Liam and Vipin Singh; Jill Dickinson; Ian, Tiffany, and Alex McFadden; Harrison and Kirsten Mills: thank you for helping me honor his legacy. To my late father, Burton Sternoff: thank you for bestowing a love a books and silly jokes!

Finally, I am profoundly grateful for my growing community at Vibrant Blue Oils. Thank you for sharing your hearts, your time, your energy, your personal stories, and your brilliance. I am inspired by all of you.

For the complete, extensive bibliography with up-to-date references, go to
www.boostthebrainbook.com/resources.

Agah, Shahram, Amir Mehdi Taleb, Reyhane Moeini, Narjes Gorji, and Hajar
    Nikbakht. "Cumin Extract for Symptom Control in Patients with Irritable
    Bowel Syndrome: A Case Series." *Middle East Journal of Digestive*
    Diseases 5, no. 4 (October 2013): 217–22. https://www.ncbi.nlm.nih.gov/
    pubmed/24829694.
Agatonovic-Kustrin, Snezana, Ella Kustrin, and David W. Morton.
    "Essential Oils and Functional Herbs for Healthy Aging." *Neural*
    Regeneration Research 14, no. 3 (March 2019): 441–45. https://doi
    .org/10.4103/1673-5374.245467.
Alma, Mehmet Hakki, Siegfried Nitz, Hubert Kollmannsberger, Metin Diğrak,
    Fatih Tuncay Efe, and Necmettin Yilmaz. "Chemical Composition and
    Antimicrobial Activity of the Essential Oils from the Gum of Turkish
    Pistachio (*Pistacia vera* L.)." *Journal of Agricultural and Food Chemistry*
    52, no. 12 (June 2004): 3911–14. https://doi.org/10.1021/jf040014e.
Alqareer, Athbi, Asma Alyahya, and Lars Andersson. "The Effect of Clove
    and Benzocaine Versus Placebo as Topical Anesthetics." *Journal of*
    Dentistry 34, no. 10 (November 2006): 747–50. https://doi.org/10.1016/j
    .jdent.2006.01.009.
Antonucci, Nicola, Dietrich Klinghardt, Stefania Pacini, and Marco Ruggiero.
    "Tailoring the Ruggiero-Klinghardt Protocol to Immunotherapy of Autism."
    American Journal of Immunology 14, no. 1 (January 2018): 34–41. https://
    doi.org/10.3844/ajisp.2018.34.41.
Ayaz, Muhammad, Abdul Sadiq, Muhammad Junaid, Farhat Ullah,
    Fazal Subhan, and Jawad Ahmed. "Neuroprotective and Anti-aging
    Potentials of Essential Oils from Aromatic and Medicinal Plants." *Frontiers*
    in Aging Neuroscience 9 (May 30, 2017): 168. https://dx.doi
    .org/10.3389%2Ffnagi.2017.00168.
Boukhris, Maher, Mohamed Bouaziz, Ines Feki, Hedya Jemai, Abdelfattah
    El Feki, and Sami Sayadi. "Hypoglycemic and Antioxidant Effects of Leaf
    Essential Oil of *Pelargonium graveolens* L'Hér. in Alloxan-Induced Diabetic
    Rats." *Lipids in Health and Disease* 11, no. 81 (June 26, 2012): 81. https://doi
    .org/10.1186/1476-511x-11-81.

Bradley, Belinda F., Nicola J. Starkey, S. L. Brown, and Robert Lea. "The Effects of Prolonged Rose Odor Inhalation in Two Animal Models of Anxiety." *Physiology & Behavior* 92, no. 5 (December 2007): 931–38. https://doi.org/10.1016/j.physbeh.2007.06.023.

Campbell-McBride, Natasha. *Gut and Psychology Syndrome: Natural Treatment for Autism, Dyspraxia, A.D.D., Dyslexia, A.D.H.D., Depression, Schizophrenia.* London: Medinform, 2004.

Chaudhuri, Joydeep. "Blood Brain Barrier and Infection." *Medical Science Monitor* 6, no. 6 (November–December 2000): 1213–22. https://pubmed.ncbi.nlm.nih.gov/11208482/.

Cherkasova, Marlya V., and Lily Hechtman. "Neuroimaging in Attention-Deficit Hyperactivity Disorder: Beyond the Frontostriatal Circuitry." *The Canadian Journal of Psychiatry* 54, no. 10, (October 2009): 651–64. https://doi.org/10.1177/070674370905401002.

Fischer, Tobias W., Ralph M. Trüeb, Gabriella Hänggi, Marcello Innocenti, and Peter Elsner. "Topical Melatonin for Treatment of Androgenetic Alopecia." *International Journal of Trichology* 4, no. 4 (October 2012): 236–45. https://doi.org/10.4103/0974-7753.111199.

Fox, Michelle, Ellie Krueger, Lauren Putterman, and Robert Schroeder. "The Effect of Peppermint on Memory Performance." *Journal of Advanced Student Science (JASS)*, University of Wisconsin-School of Medicine and Public Health, Department of Neuroscience, and University of Wisconsin-School of Education, Department of Kinesiology (Spring 2012). http://jass.neuro.wisc.edu/2012/01/Lab%20603%20Group%205%20The%20Effect%20of%20Peppermint%20on%20Memory%20Performance.pdf.

Friedmann, Terry S. "Attention Deficit and Hyperactivity Disorder (ADHD)." *Semantic Scholar*, Corpus ID: 51436208 (2002). https://www.semanticscholar.org/paper/ATTENTION-DEFICIT-AND-HYPERACTIVITY-DISORDER-(-ADHD-Friedmann/c24c35b7ceea6a3e09ea2ca773b354eea318e6c2.

Fu, Yujie, Yuangang Zu, Liyan Chen, Xiaoguang Shi, Zhe Wang, Su Sun, and Thomas Efferth. "Antimicrobial Activity of Clove and Rosemary Essential Oils Alone and in Combination." *Phytotherapy Research* 21, no. 10 (October 2007): 989–94. https://doi.org/10.1002/ptr.2179.

Garabadu, Debapriya, Ankit Shah, Sanjay Singh, and Sairam Krishnamurthy. "Protective Effect of Eugenol Against Restraint Stress-Induced Gastrointestinal Dysfunction: Potential Use in Irritable Bowel Syndrome." *Pharmaceutical Biology* 53, no. 7, 968–74. https://doi.org/10.3109/13880209.2014.950674.

Georas, Steve N., and Fariba Rezaee. "Epithelial Barrier Function: At the Frontline of Asthma Immunology and Allergic Airway Inflammation." *The Journal of Allergy and Clinical Immunology* 134, no. 3 (September 1, 2014): 509–20. https://doi.org/10.1016/j.jaci.2014.05.049.

Goleman, Daniel. "Brain's Design Emerges as a Key to Emotions." *New York Times*, August 15, 1989. https://www.nytimes.com/1989/08/15/science/brain-s-design-emerges-as-a-key-to-emotions.html.

Habib, Navaz. *Activate Your Vagus Nerve*. Berkeley: Ulysses Press, 2019.

Han, Xuesheng, Tory L. Parker, and Jeff Dorsett. "An Essential Oil Blend Significantly Modulates Immune Responses and the Cell Cycle in Human Cell Cultures." *Cogent Biology* 3, no. 1 (June 2017). https://doi.org/10.1080/23312025.2017.1340112.

Hay, Louise. *You Can Heal Your Life*. Carlsbad, CA: Hay House, 2004.

He, Wei, Xiaoyu Wang, Hong Shi, Hongyan Shang, Liang Li, Xiang-Hong Jing, and Bing Zhu. "Auricular Acupuncture and Vagal Regulation." *Evidence-Based Complementary and Alternative Medicine*, Article ID 786839 (November 27, 2012). https://doi.org/10.1155/2012/786839.

Herz, Rachel S. "Do Scents Affect People's Moods or Work Performance?" *Scientific American*, November 11, 2002. https://www.scientificamerican.com/article/do-scents-affect-peoples/.

Hotta, Mariko, Rieko Nakata, Michiko Katsukawa, Kazuyuki Hori, Saori Takahashi, and Inoue Hiroyasu. "Carvacrol, a Component of Thyme Oil, Activates PPARα and γ and Suppresses COX-2 Expression." *Journal of Lipid Research* 51, no. 1 (January 2010): 132–39. https://doi.org/10.1194/jlr.m900255-jlr200.

Kharrazian, Datis. *Why Isn't My Brain Working?: A Revolutionary Understanding of Brain Decline and Effective Strategies to Recover Your Brain's Health*. Carlsbad, CA: Elephant Press, 2013.

Kiecolt-Glaser, Janice K., Jennifer E. Graham-Engeland, William B. Malarkey, Kyle Porter, Stanley Lemeshow, and Ronald Glaser. "Olfactory Influences on Mood and Autonomic, Endocrine, and Immune Function." *Psychoneuroendocrinology* 33, no. 3 (April 2008): 328–39. https://doi.org/10.1016/j.psyneuen.2007.11.015.

Kim, Yong-Guy, Jin-Hyung Lee, Giyeon Gwon, Soon-Il Kim, Jae Gyu Park, and Jintae Lee. "Essential Oils and Eugenols Inhibit Biofilm Formation and the Virulence of *Escherichia coli* O157:H7." *Scientific Reports* 6, Article ID 36377 (November 3, 2016). https://doi.org/10.1038/srep36377.

Klinghardt, Dietrich, and Amelie Schmeer-Maurer. Mentalfeld-Techniken—
    Ganz Praktisch: 20 Methoden für Selbsthilfe und Heilung. Kirchzarten,
    Germany: VAK Verlags, 2011.
Komori, T., R. Fujiwara, M. Tanida, J. Nomura, and M. M. Yokoyama. "Effects
    of Citrus Fragrance on Immune Function and Depressive States."
    Neuroimmunomodulation 2, no. 3 (May–June 1995): 174–80. https://doi
    .org/10.1159/000096889.
Kong, Jian, Jiliang Fang, Joel Park, Shaoyuan Li, and Pei-Jing Rong.
    "Treating Depression with Transcutaneous Auricular Vagus Nerve
    Stimulation: State of the Art and Future Perspectives." Frontiers in
    Psychiatry (February 5, 2018). https://doi.org/10.3389/fpsyt.2018.00020.
Lang, Dr. Janet. "Balancing Female Horomones Naturally." [Lecture.] Seattle:
    May, 2010.
Lang, Sidney B., Andrew A. Marino, Garry Berkovic, Marjorie Fowler,
    and Kenneth D. Abreo. "Piezoelectricity in the Human Pineal Gland."
    Bioelectrochemistry and Bioenergetics 41, no. 2 (December 1996): 191–95.
    https://doi.org/10.1016/S0302-4598(96)05147-1.
Lee, Jin-Hyung, Yong-Guy Kim, and Jintae Lee. "Carvacrol-Rich Oregano
    Oil and Thymol-Rich Thyme Red Oil Inhibit Biofilm Formation and
    the Virulence of Uropathogenic Escherichia coli. Journal of Applied
    Microbiology 123, no. 6 (December 2017): 1420–28. https://doi.org/10.1111/
    jam.13602.
Li, Yuan, Xiongfeng Fu, Xin Ma, Shijie Geng, Xuemei Jiang, Qichun Huang,
    Caihong Hu, and Xinyan Han. "Intestinal Microbiome-Metabolome
    Responses to Essential Oils in Piglets." Frontiers in Microbiology 9
    (August 28, 2018): 1988. https://dx.doi.org/10.3389%2Ffmicb.2018.01988.
Liu, Ai-Dong, Guo-Hong Cai, Yan-Yan Wei, Jian-Ping Yu, Jing Chen,
    Jing Yang, Xin Wang, Yin-Wei Che, Jian-Zong Chen, and Sheng-Xi
    Wu. "Anxiolytic Effect of Essential Oils of Salvia miltiorrhiza in Rats."
    International Journal of Clinical and Experimental Medicine 8, no. 8
    (November 2015): 12756–64. http://www.ncbi.nlm.nih.gov/pmc/articles/
    pmc4612874/.
Louis, Janelle. "Adverse Childhood Experiences: A Hidden Cause of
    Depression & Chronic Disease." Naturopathic Doctor News & Review,
    March 4, 2019. https://ndnr.com/anxietydepressionmental-health/adverse-
    childhood-experiences-a-hidden-cause-of-depression-chronic-disease/.
Lv, Xiao Nan, Huan Jing Zhang, and Chi-Meng Tzeng. "Aromatherapy
    and the Central Nerve System (CNS): Therapeutic Mechanism and Its
    Associated Genes." Current Drug Targets 14, no. 8 (July 2013): 872–79.
    https://doi.org/10.2174/1389450111314080007.

Matsukawa, Mutsumi, Masato Imada, Toyotaka Murakami, Shin Aizawa, and Takaaki Sato. "Rose Odor Can Innately Counteract Predator Odor." *Brain Research* 1381 (March 24, 2011): 117–23. https://doi.org/10.1016/j.brainres.2011.01.053.

Morgan, L. Lloyd, Santosh Kesari, and Devra Lee Davis. "Why Children Absorb More Microwave Radiation than Adults: The Consequences." *Journal of Microscopy and Ultrastructure* 2, no. 4 (December 2014): 197–204. https://doi.org/10.1016/j.jmau.2014.06.005.

Moss, Mark, and Lorraine Oliver. "Plasma 1,8-Cineole Correlates with Cognitive Performance Following Exposure to Rosemary Essential Oil Aroma." *Therapeutic Advances in Psychopharmacology* 2, no. 3 (June 2012): 103–13. https://doi.org/10.1177/2045125312436573.

Nahman-Averbuch, Hadas, Elliot Sprecher, Giris Jacob, and David Yarnitsky. "The Relationships Between Parasympathetic Function and Pain Perception: The Role of Anxiety." *Pain Practice* 16, no. 8 (November 2016): 1064–72. https://doi.org/10.1111/papr.12407.

Nazzaro, Filomena, Florinda Fratianni, Laura De Martino, Raffaele Coppola, and Vincenzo De Feo. "Effect of Essential Oils on Pathogenic Bacteria." *Pharmaceuticals (Basel)* 6, no. 12 (December 2013): 1451–74. https://doi.org/10.3390/ph6121451.

Negoias, Simona, Ilona Croy, Johannes Gerber, S. Puschmann, Katja Petrowski, Peter Joraschky, and Thomas Hummel. "Reduced Olfactory Bulb Volume and Olfactory Sensitivity in Patients with Acute Major Depression." *Neuroscience* 169, no. 1 (August 11, 2010): 415–21. https://doi.org/10.1016/j.neuroscience.2010.05.012.

Nicoll, Roger A., and Daniel V. Madison. "General Anesthetics Hyperpolarize Neurons in the Vertebrate Central Nervous System." *Science* 217, no. 4564 (September 10, 1982): 1055–57. https://doi.org/10.1126/science.7112112.

Pavlov, Valentin A., and Kevin J. Tracey. "Neural Circuitry and Immunity." *Immunologic Research* 63, no. 0 (December 2015): 38–57. https://doi.org/10.1007/s12026-015-8718-1.

Peres, Mario Fernando Prieto, Eliova Zukerman, Fabiano da Cunha Tanuri, F. R. Moreira, and Jose Cipolla-Neto. "Melatonin, 3 Mg, Is Effective for Migraine Prevention." *Neurology* 63, no. 4 (August 24, 2004): 757. https://doi.org/10.1212/01.WNL.0000134653.35587.24.

Pizzorno, Joseph E. *The Toxin Solution: How Hidden Poisons in the Air, Water, Food, and Products We Use Are Destroying Our Health—and What We Can Do to Fix It.* New York: HarperOne, 2017.

Qin, Bolin, Kiran S. Panickar, and Richard A. Anderson. "Cinnamon: Potential Role in the Prevention of Insulin Resistance, Metabolic Syndrome, and Type 2 Diabetes." *Journal of Diabetes Science and Technology* 4, no. 3 (May 2010): 685–93. https://doi.org/10.1177/193229681000400324.

Reiter, Russel J., Du-Xian Tan, Ahmet Korkmaz, and Lorena Fuentes-Broto. "Drug-Mediated Ototoxicity and Tinnitus: Alleviation with Melatonin." *Journal of Physiology and Pharmacology* 62, no. 2 (April 1, 2011): 151–57. http://www.jpp.krakow.pl/journal/archive/04_11/pdf/151_04_11_article.pdf.

Samsel, Anthony, and Stephanie Seneff. "Glyphosate, Pathways to Modern Diseases III: Manganese, Neurological Diseases, and Associated Pathologies." *Surgical Neurology International* 6 (March 24, 2015): 45. https://doi.org/10.4103/2152-7806.153876.

Sapolsky, Robert M. *Why Zebras Don't Get Ulcers: The Acclaimed Guide to Stress, Stress-Related Diseases, and Coping.* 3rd ed. New York: Henry Holt, 2004.

Seneff, Stephanie. "Sulfate Deficiency in Neurological Disease Following Aluminum and Glyphosate Exposure." Webinar presented on June 2, 2015, hosted by Jessica Sherman. https://people.csail.mit.edu/seneff/2015/SeneffJune2_2015.pdf.

Seol, Geun Hee, Hyun Soo Shim, Pill-Joo Kim, Hea Kyung Moon, Ki-Ho Lee, Insop Shim, Suk Hyo Suh, and Sun Seek Min. "Antidepressant-like Effect of *Salvia sclarea* Is Explained by Modulation of Dopamine Activities in Rats." *Journal of Ethnopharmacology* 130, no. 1 (July 6, 2010): 187–90. https://doi.org/10.1016/j.jep.2010.04.035.

Simon Fraser University. "Understanding How the Blood-Brain Barrier Is Breached in Bacterial Meningitis." *Infection Control Today*, October 5, 2016. https://www.infectioncontroltoday.com/view/understanding-how-blood-brain-barrier-breached-bacterial-meningitis.

Stewart, David. *The Chemistry of Essential Oils Made Simple: God's Love Manifest in Molecules.* Marble Hill, MO: Care Publications, 2005.

Su, Shulan, Jinao Duan, Ting Chen, Xiaochen Huang, Erxin Shang, Li Yu, Kaifeng Wei, et al. "Frankincense and Myrrh Suppress Inflammation via Regulation of the Metabolic Profiling and the MAPK Signaling Pathway." *Scientific Reports* 5, Article ID 13668 (September 2, 2015). https://doi.org/10.1038/srep13668.

Surette, Marc E. "The Science Behind Dietary Omega-3 Fatty Acids." *Canadian Medical Association Journal* 178, no. 2 (January 15, 2008): 177–80. https://doi.org/10.1503/cmaj.071356.

Takeda, Ai, Emiko Watanuki, and Sachiyo Koyama. "Effects of Inhalation Aromatherapy on Symptoms of Sleep Disturbance in the Elderly with Dementia." *Evidence-Based Complementary and Alternative Medicine* 4, Article ID 1902807 (March 23, 2017): 1–7. https://doi.org/10.1155/2017/1902807.

Talpur, N., Bobby Echard, C. Ingram, Debasis Bagchi, and Harry G. Preuss. "Effects of a Novel Formulation of Essential Oils on Glucose-Insulin Metabolism in Diabetic and Hypertensive Rats: A Pilot Study." *Diabetes, Obesity and Metabolism* 7, no. 2 (March 2005): 193–99. https://doi.org/10.1111/j.1463-1326.2004.00386.x.

Tamura, Hiroshi, Akihisa Takasaki, Toshiaki Taketani, Manabu Tanabe, Fumie Kizuka, Lifa Lee, Isao Tamura, et al. "The Role of Melatonin as an Antioxidant in the Follicle." *Journal of Ovarian Research* 5, no. 5 (January 26, 2012). https://doi.org/10.1186/1757-2215-5-5.

Targum, Steven D., and Norman Rosenthal. "Seasonal Affective Disorder." *Psychiatry (Edgmont)* 5, no. 5 (May 2008): 31–33: https://www.ncbi.nlm.nih.gov/pmc/articles/PMC2686645/.

Tompa, Rachel. "Tracing the Scent of Fear: Study Identifies Region of Brain Involved in Fear Response." *Hutch News Stories*, Fred Hutchinson Cancer Research Center, March 21, 2016. https://www.fredhutch.org/en/news/center-news/2016/03/fear-response-brain-region-identified.html.

VanElzakker, Michael B. "Chronic Fatigue Syndrome from Vagus Nerve Infection: A Psychoneuroimmunological Hypothesis." *Medical Hypotheses* 81, no. 3 (September 2013): 414–23. https://doi.org/10.1016/j.mehy.2013.05.034.

Waring, Rosemary H. "Report on Absorption of Magnesium Sulfate (Epsom Salts) Across the Skin." Epsom Salt Council, accessed October 7, 2019. https://www.epsomsaltcouncil.org/wp-content/uploads/2015/10/report_on_absorption_of_magnesium_sulfate.pdf.

Wierenga, Christina E., Amanda Bischoff-Grethe, A. James Melrose, Zoe Irvine, Laura Torres, Ursula F. Bailer, Alan Simmons, Julie L. Fudge, Samuel M. McClure, Alice V. Ely, and Walter H. Kaye. "Hunger Does Not Motivate Reward in Women Remitted from Anorexia Nervosa." *Biological Psychiatry* 77, no. 7 (April 1, 2015): 642–52. https://doi.org/10.1016/j.biopsych.2014.09.024.

Wolfe, David. "This Essential Oil Stops Sugar Cravings and Helps You Lose Weight." DavidWolfe.com, accessed October 7, 2020. https://www.david-wolfe.com/essential-oils-stops-sugar-cravings-lose-weight/.

Woo, Chern Chiuh, Alan Prem Kumar, Gautam Sethi, and Kwong Huat Benny Tan. "Thymoquinone: Potential Cure for Inflammatory Disorders and Cancer." *Biochemical Pharmacology* 83, no. 4 (February 15, 2012): 443–51. https://doi.org/10.1016/j.bcp.2011.09.029.

Worwood, Valerie Ann. *Aromatherapy for the Soul: Healing the Spirit with Fragrance and Essential Oils.* Novato, CA: New World Library, 1999.

Zheng, Qun, Zi-Xian Chen, Meng-Bei Xu, Xiao-Li Zhou, Yue-Yue Huang, Guo-Qing Zheng, and Yan Wang. "Borneol, a Messenger Agent, Improves Central Nervous System *Drug Delivery* Through Enhancing Blood-Brain Barrier Permeability: A Preclinical Systematic Review and Meta-analysis." Drug Delivery 25, no. 1 (November 2018): 1617–33. https://doi.org/10.1080/10717544.2018.1486471.

frankincense, 147, 156, 161, 176, 177, 183–84, 188, 191, 201, 203
free radicals, 53
Friedmann, Terry, 102, 202
frontal lobe, 95–96, 98

G

GABA (gamma-aminobutyric acid), 7, 36, 117, 120
gallbladder, 54, 75, 79, 174–75, 179, 180
Gattefossé, René-Maurice, 156
geranium oil, 176, 185
GERD (gastroesophageal reflux disease), 28–29, 55
ghrelin, 123, 130
ginger, 178, 187, 191
glial cells, 65, 66, 150, 151
glutamate, 121
glutathione, 160, 171
glymphatic system, 64–65, 66
glyphosate, 56, 60, 197
grapefruit oil, 176, 178, 179, 187
gut health, 31, 55, 152, 158, 159, 188–89, 199

H

Habib, Navaz, 47
hair loss, 55–56, 125
Hay, Louise, 203
health, five keys to
benefits of, 194–95
daily implementation of, 194–95
detailed description of, 169–93
list of, 167
heartburn, 37, 55
heart health, 32, 37, 54
heavy metals, 38, 54, 77, 80, 143, 197–98

helichrysum oil, 154, 176, 179, 189
Herz, Rachel, 113
hippocampus, 88, 111, 113
Hirsch, Alan R., 129
histamine, 158, 189
holy basil oil, 191
homeostasis, 125
hormones
cell receptors and, 133–34
definition of, 123
imbalance in, 127, 129, 132–33, 175
insulin resistance and, 92
role of, 123
weight and, 129–31
HPA (hypothalamic-pituitary-adrenal) axis, 107, 108–9
HRV (heart rate variability), 47
hydration, 201
hypothalamus, 91, 108, 109, 111, 123, 125–27, 129, 183–84, 185
Hypothalamus Blend, 184
hyssop oil, 191

I

IBS (irritable bowel syndrome), 9, 27, 28, 36, 46, 180
immune system
body temperature and, 162
brain and, 150
importance of, 136, 149
melatonin and, 53
parasympathetic state and, 29
supporting, 149–50, 152–54, 156–62, 187
infections, fighting, 29, 162
inflammation
acute, 137
Anti-Inflammatory Blend, 187

noradrenaline (norepinephrine), 118, 132
nutmeg oil, 178, 191

O

oil pulling, 3–4, 70
olfactory bulb, 12
olfactory epithelium, 12
omega-3 fatty acids, 145–46
orange oil, 44
oregano oil, 7, 93, 191, 200
oxygen, 82, 85–86

P

pain
  inflammation and, 139
  vagus nerve and, 30, 36
palmarosa oil, 176
pancreas, 130, 132, 184–85
panic attacks, 37, 43, 98, 107, 112
parasites, 39
parasympathetic nervous system
  activation of, 26, 76
  role of, 25–26
parasympathetic state
  benefits of, 28–34
  definition of, 26
  healing and, 26
  Parasympathetic Blend, 169
  quiz, 27
  shifting into, 169–71
  vagus nerve and, 25–26
Parkinson's disease, 1, 51, 53, 58, 60, 85, 91, 137, 150
patchouli oil, 184
peppermint oil, 9, 64, 68, 70, 79, 129, 147, 157, 176, 178, 186

peptide YY, 130, 131
phenylpropanoids, 93, 133
pineal gland, 51, 56, 58–61, 172
pine oil, 184
piperine, 86
pituitary gland, 108, 109, 126
Pizzorno, Joseph, 78, 89
PMS, 77, 119, 125
prefrontal cortex, 95–97, 100–102, 201
protein digestion, 160–61
PTSD (post-traumatic stress disorder), 33, 41, 85, 97, 101, 109, 127
pulse points, applying essential oils to, 14

R

ravensara oil, 191
red mandarin oil, 184
re-toxification, 80
Roman chamomile oil, 9
rose geranium oil, 172, 185
rosemary oil, 9, 183, 186, 191
rose oil, 8, 118, 185, 203
Ruggiero, Marco, 40

S

safety precautions, 18
Sapolsky, Robert M., 41
Seneff, Stephanie, 56
serotonin, 117, 119–20
sesquiterpenes, 85–86, 177, 183
sexual health, 32
shift-work disorder, 53
SIBO (small intestine bacterial overgrowth), 27, 28, 36

trauma
blood-brain barrier and, 143
hormones and, 126
parasympathetic state and, 33
vagus nerve toxicity and, 40–44
Treg cells (regulatory T-cells), 161
tryptophan, 52, 60, 117
tumor necrosis factor (TNF), 146

U

ulcers, 29, 55, 107, 191, 199
uterus, 32, 75

V

vagal tone
definition of, 45, 46
effects of, 46–47
measuring, 47
vagus nerve
acetylcholine and, 120–21
diagram of, 24
importance of, 22–23, 35
inflammation and, 146
neck congestion and, 69
parasympathetic state and,
25–26, 28–34
role of, 23, 25
stimulation, 45–48
supporting, 178–79
vagus nerve dysfunction (toxicity)
causes of, 37–44
effects of, 35–36
prevalence of, 35
symptoms of, 36–37
VanElzakker, Michael, 39
vanilla, 121
vetiver oil, 202
viral infections, 39
vitex berry oil, 176

W

water, 201
weight
hormones and, 129–31
insulin resistance and, 91, 92
vagus nerve and, 33, 37
Wells, Katie, 70
Worwood, Valerie Ann, 5

Y

ylang-ylang oil, 118, 121, 176, 178

Text copyright © 2021 by Jodi Sternoff Cohen
Illustrations copyright © 2021 by Penguin Random House LLC

All rights reserved.
Published in the United States by Ten Speed Press, an imprint of Random House, a division of Penguin Random House LLC, New York.
www.tenspeed.com

Ten Speed Press and the Ten Speed Press colophon are registered trademarks of Penguin Random House LLC.

Library of Congress Control Number: 2020942363

Hardcover ISBN: 978-1-9848-5860-3
eBook ISBN: 978-1-9848-5861-0

Front cover graphic and page 42 graphic by Roy Migabon
Image on pages ii–iii, 20–21, 164–165, and 206–207 by Stock.Adobe.com
Image on page vi by Nattika/Shutterstock.com
Image on pages xi, 122, and 163 by Pevuna/Shutterstock.com
Image on page xii by OlgaOtto/Shutterstock.com
Image on page 49 by Ohhlanla/Shutterstock.com
Image on page 62 by Marianna Kara/Shutterstock.com
Image on page 94 by EKramar/Shutterstock.com
Image on page 114, 148, 155, 166–167, and 196–197 by Flaffy/Shutterstock.com
Image on page 128 by Zamurovic Brothers/Shutterstock.com
Image on page 135 by Nella/Shutterstock.com
Author photo by Lisi Wolf

Printed in the U.S.A.

10 9 8 7 6 5 4 3

First Edition